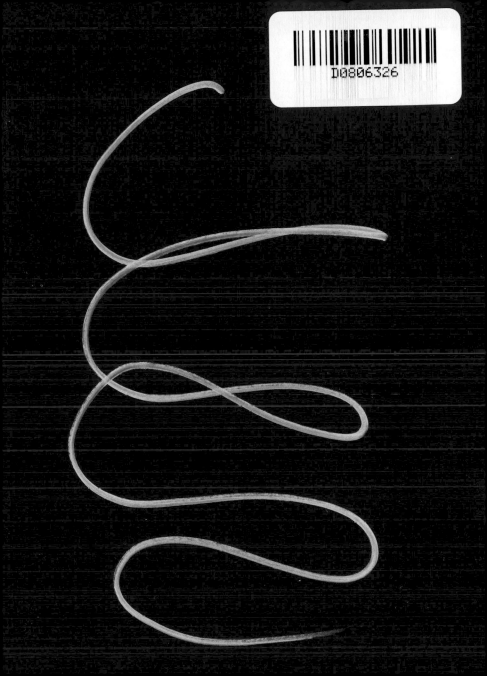

THE VOICE OF SILENCE

THE VOICE OF SILENCE

A LIFE OF LOVE,
HEALING AND INSPIRATION

Oonagh Shanley-Toffolo

RIDER

LONDON · SYDNEY · AUCKLAND · JOHANNESBURG

1 3 5 7 9 10 8 6 4 2

First published in 2002 by Rider,
an imprint of Ebury Press, Random House,
20 Vauxhall Bridge Road, London SW1V 2SA

Random House Australia (Pty) Limited
20 Alfred Street, Milsons Point, Sydney,
New South Wales 2061, Australia

Random House New Zealand Limited
18 Poland Road, Glenfield,
Auckland 10, New Zealand

Random House South Africa (Pty) Limited
Endulini, 5A Jubilee Road,
Parktown 2193, South Africa

The Random House Group Limited Reg. No. 954009

Papers used by Rider are natural, recyclable products made from wood
grown in sustainable forests.

Printed and bound by Mackays of Chatham plc, Kent

A CIP catalogue record for this book is available from the British Library

ISBN 0-7126-1445-1

The author and publisher are grateful to the Catholic Truth Society for permission
to quote Jerome Vereb CP on Ignatius Spencer; Mrs H M Davies Will Trust for
permission to quote from 'Leisure' by W H Davies; Dover Publications for the
quotation from *Gitanjali* by Rabindranath Tagore (Dover, 2000); and Penguin for the
quotation from *The Essential Rumi*, trans. Coleman Barks (Arkana, 1999). Every
effort has been made to trace all copyright holders, but if any have been overlooked the
publishers will be pleased to make the necessary arrangement at the first opportunity.

To my beloved Joseph.

'Winter is gone,
the flowers have appeared in the land.'
– Solomon

CONTENTS

CONTENTS

GRATITUDE TO:

The Divine Author of Love.

My creative and talented editor, Judith Kendra, who wove her silken threads to embellish *The Voice of Silence* after resurrecting it.

Laura Morris, my literary agent, who supported me and this book with so much generosity.

Selina Walker who guided the Voice and found the bearer, Laura Morris, who embraced it with love.

Amelia Thorpe, for her charismatic welcome, and to all those at Rider/Random House who had any involvement in the making of *The Voice of Silence*.

Gayle Warwick, whose fidelity and friendship rescued me in my darkest hour.

Gael Kennedy who, since our Parisian days, has kept our friendship kindled with fun faxes and measured wisdom.

Elaine Williams, Angel of the Morning, and my own healer.

Sister Mairead Leonard, poor servant of the Mother of God, with whom I have shared my love of Mary, Our Divine Mother.

Rosario de Kling who also loves Mary and believed in my dream.

Vicki Barker whose voice awakens America and who gave Joseph and myself much pleasure.

The daughters and sons, sisters and brothers adopted spiritually along the way.

The children of all nations reaching out with love.

Many other names are etched in the brightest stars. I shall keep you all in the light of Christ's love.

A STRONG WOMAN
vs A WOMAN OF STRENGTH

A strong woman works out every day to keep her body
in shape . . .
but a woman of strength builds relationships to keep her
soul in shape.
A strong woman isn't afraid of anything . . .
but a woman of strength shows courage in the midst of
fear.
A strong woman won't let anyone get the better of
her . . .
but the woman of strength gives the best of herself to
everyone.
A strong woman makes mistakes and avoids the same
in the future . . .
A woman of strength realises life's mistakes can also be
unexpected blessings, and capitalises on them.
A strong woman wears a look of confidence on her face
. . . but a woman of strength wears grace.
A strong woman has faith that she is strong enough for
the journey . . .
but the woman of strength has faith that it is in the
journey that she will become strong.

(Author unknown)

FOREWORD

From as early as I can remember – please do not laugh – I dreamed of being a martyr in China. I used to sit on the kitchen floor and look at the willow pattern plates on my mother's dresser and dream. My father would tease me and say, 'Yes, you will have a Chinese martyrdom – of pinpricks!' How prophetic. Years later I would discover the wisdom of acupuncture and be one of the first students to gain entry to China after the Cultural Revolution.

Dreams have always been an important part of my life. I have tried to watch them rise to the surface and follow them rather than doing the things I thought I should, or that other people thought I ought. In this way there is more hope of being fulfilled and becoming a free spirit, rather than being constantly pulled in a thousand different directions, none of which may be true to your own heart.

Dreams, and more dreams, led me to become a nun, to train as a nurse in Dublin, to spend time in France and to leave for India to care for the poor (I long ago learned to define poverty as a lack of love, whether it be spiritual, emotional or physical). They also directed me to Paris, my true spiritual home, a city where I have lived and loved – and where I hope one day to die.

Convent life was an excellent grounding in discipline and

humility, which were instilled into us over a long period of time by gentle and convincing religious. We were still in our formative years and had not, as yet, acquired too many bad habits! The training in monastic observance taught us the value of the more important things in life: to be calm in stressful situations and to remain in a state of peace, which is all about prayer. This spiritual path turned me into the person I became during my twenty years of living in a wonderful community of people who were all striving for perfection. However, the journey did not come to an end when I left the convent: it continues to this day.

Along the route I was given charge of the ex-King Edward VIII, who needed an experienced nurse to make his last months on earth more tolerable. I know the world and history have judged the Duke of Windsor and found him wanting as a public man, but I knew him as a private one, and came to see that his courage in illness was as staunch as his courage in love. I was also struck by his humility. He was a man before his time, whom the Establishment rejected. It was not then ready to hear about love and to shatter the rigid mould of the monarchy which did not allow its children to breathe freely.

Another dream I had was to study midwifery. This was realised in the many mothers and babies I cared for along the way, and finally brought into my life Diana, Princess of Wales – a mother to her sons, and of the unloved wherever and whoever they were.

Both the Duke of Windsor and the Princess of Wales had the

courage of their convictions, dared to be different and to live their own truth. Somehow it was my destiny to share in the lives of these two extraordinary and unusual souls who lived and died only twenty-five years apart.

A quest for self-discovery, the pursuit of love in all its forms, and the recognition and development of my capacity for healing have been clear themes of my journey. At first, in my innocence, I thought healers did not need to study or to learn but simply needed miraculous powers, but soon I learned that though one may have an aptitude, one does need to study techniques and practise skills to be useful. More than anything, one needs to be 'wounded' oneself in order to truly help others.

My greatest lessons in compassion came from my own illnesses and being out of control of my own bodily functions. I often felt like Job on his dunghill: Satan challenged God and asked permission to test Job, who had been blessed with good fortune. God agreed and Job was sent every sort of affliction but somehow never lost his faith and his capacity to love. Pain and illness (with their accompanying frustrations and isolation) taught me to open to the blessings of love, and to be able to receive. As I discovered, receiving can be much harder than giving. I also found that recreation, laughter, travel and curiosity can fire the heart. Singing and feeling joy are important as well. As Shakespeare said, 'He who sings prays twice.'

My surname, Shanley, means 'Old Warrior', from the Gaelic *Seanlaoch,* and my own path through life has often felt like that of a warrior on a mission. I have been led into arenas I never imagined as a child, a million light years from the dreams I had in my mother's kitchen in Ireland. But through it all, I have tried to turn towards the joy, the love and the excitement of life that is available to us all. Along the way there have been pockets of pain and peace in unexpected, secret places, but I have found that the written word which speaks of the soul's longing will take us beyond our pain into the deepest, most peaceful part of our spirit. Of all poems, perhaps the Song of Solomon is the most evocative of fulfilment, both spiritual and sensual. Worldly satisfactions are fine in themselves but perfect love and fulfilment are found elsewhere, usually in silence.

'Arise my love, my dove, my beautiful one and come . . . Winter is gone. The flowers have appeared in the land.'

Each day can be a pursuit, a discovery . . . Your life, my life, our lives are surely for living and loving – and for being happy.

CHAPTER 1

EARLY CHILDHOOD IN IRELAND

A child's education is laid down twenty years
before birth – Shakespeare

My Irish childhood was a magical experience filled with fairies, fairy tales and the natural world. In Spring the fields were blessed to bring forth a good harvest, on May Day we went out at dawn to wash our faces in the morning dew. Summer brought the cuckoo song, the corncrake and all the other beautiful sounds of nature. My father would sing the old Irish air:

> The Bee, the Bat, the Butterfly
> The Cuckoo and the Swallow
> The Corncrake put out its beak
> To wish them all Good Morrow!

The Autumn produced golden harvests, balmy evenings, the swallows leaving and wild geese flying in perfect formation. The Winter was a time for gathering around the fire, reading or being read to, singing and playing the flute. Two first cousins who were brilliant violinists used to play for us on feast days and for celebrations. Music was very important to my father, who listened to his favourite records on the gramophone and with great satisfaction around the blazing turf fire on a Sunday afternoon.

It was a simple childhood in the Leitrim countryside, near Mohill. Leitrim is a small and lovely county which lies in the north-west of Ireland between Longford and Sligo with the beautiful River Shannon running through it. The river held a great fascination for me because at a certain village there was a drawbridge which I used to cross with trepidation, fearing the bridge would go up and engulf me and my bicycle. But as a fifteen-year-old much of the scenic beauty was lost on me – arriving at my destination was becoming the main thing.

I was born on Mary's Day, the 15th of August at twelve noon and to my father I was a child sent from Heaven. At my birth when I was placed in my mother's arms she took one look at me and said, 'Who is going to look after this child?' (I was sickly and she had already borne several other children), and she handed me straight back into the arms of my father. From that moment we were bonded for life. I was very fragile and was not expected to live, and it was my father who trod the floorboards at night comforting me. I am told I was a difficult baby, and when taken to church two days later I pulled the roof down with my screams. My godfather said, 'All the devils have gone out of her with that screaming.'

Now, with my present knowledge, I would say the screaming opened my heart chakra. I was so fragile that my father elected not to have me vaccinated.

I was named Agnes Mary but my godfather, Harry Faughman, who was only seventeen at the time, said, 'No, we must call her by her Gaelic name, Oonagh.' Oonagh! A name satisfying to pronounce – and satisfying for a child to write, with its big, round Os. Years later I learned that the O is a symbol of eternity (the first sound in the mystic 'Om') and I thank Harry for a name I cherish. Later my husband, Joseph Toffolo, would daily pronounce the great 'Om' in exercising his voice before singing.

My mother was nineteen and my father twenty-one when they married. It was a love match. There was great harmony between them and he always went with her to buy her hats and shoes. He never left the house without bidding her goodbye with a kiss and saying 'I'm going now in the name of God.' My mother was very hard-working, quick and creative. She was a trained needlewoman and made all our clothes. My father was called 'the philanthropist' and he was my inspiration. Now looking back, I realise how fortunate we are to have good and loving parents to guide us. Tall and lean, my father had a smart appearance and was rarely seen without a hat. He was a man of firm faith, with an enlightened mind, and open-hearted with anybody who needed him, whether man, woman, child or beast. Healing was his art, which he taught me. I was enveloped and fired by his enthusiasm. He gave me the four cornerstones on which my life was built: faith in God, love of mankind, truth and compassion.

My father was a farmer with a diverse curiosity. He went to evening classes to learn cabinet-making and basket-weaving besides cultivating his land and rearing cattle, horses, pigs and every type of feathered fowl. What fascinated me was watching him grafting shoots from one fruit tree to another. His pride was an apple which he called American Beauty. I do not know if such an apple exists today but I still see its beautiful rosy skin and can remember the enjoyment of its delicious taste. In the evenings when time permitted he loved to take his gun and shoot pheasants or rabbits with his dogs following. On one occasion, when I was a small child, I saw a hawk balanced on the back of a chicken trying to lift it into the air – I ran in from the garden and told my father. At once he got his gun down from the kitchen rafters and shot the hawk off the chicken. I was thrilled and my admiration for him grew even more.

He did not like to slaughter farm animals. Farming was different in Ireland in those days. Above all, farmers were crafts-men. Labour was mainly an exchange between neighbours. The *methel* was the Gaelic word used to describe the collection of farmers and neighbours invited to help with each other's harvesting. The work finished with a good dinner and a half-barrel of Guinness, followed by music and dancing.

He loved to go to auctions, mainly to buy books and china, and to the cattle fairs to sell his livestock. His books were under lock and key, nobody dared touch them.

One day a neighbour got lockjaw while arguing with my father about a right of way through his land. Quickly, my father reached into his pocket for his handkerchief and penknife, and edged the hankie-draped penknife between the teeth of his aggressor, gently and steadily releasing the jaw. After that, there was peace and no more quarrels about land rights. Many years later, this same man's daughter developed tuberculosis and was sent to a sanatorium in Manorhamilton. My aunt, who lived there, visited Anna every day. The girl returned home to die, and one morning my mother sent me with milk and fresh eggs. Anna was sitting up in bed. Gasping for breath she wanted to give me some ribbons for my hair. I tried to arrange her pillows then suddenly her breathing stopped. Her spirit had flown – she died in my arms. I raced down the stairs to alert Anna's mother and aunt who were sipping tea in the kitchen. Her aunt, terrified that I would catch the contagion, sent me home. I wandered back over the fields thinking about Anna and where she had gone. I was nine years old.

Every night, without fail, my father and mother and who-ever was in the house joined in the recitation of the Rosary, with a long litany of the Blessed Virgin Mary and further invocations. I found the hour too long on my bare knees but one prayer I still remember. 'Jesus, Mary and Joseph, save us from a sudden and unprovided death!'

To this day the words of the Litany come to mind, its age-old chant full of mystic invocations and archetypal images: Mother of God, Mother of Divine Grace, Mother Most Pure, Virgin of Virgins, Mystical Rose, House of Gold, Tower of Ivory, Seat of Wisdom, House of David, Ark of the Covenant, Gate of Heaven, and so forth. *Pray for us* was the response to each invocation. Today, more than sixty years later, these beautiful words are a solace to my heart.

Throughout his life, my father revered his own mother and it was she who had instituted the ritual of the whole household, including any stray visitors, coming together for daily prayers. It wasn't easy to share all of their devotions; but perhaps it was fertile soil for dreams of a missionary vocation.

One day I was taken by the gypsies. My father came home to discover I was missing. However, he who knew everybody lost no time in finding the gypsy camp. There I was, enthralled by the many objects of curiosity – the monkeys, the birds, the animals. The gypsies said they had found me wandering so my father gave them a silver coin, took me on his shoulders and carried me home and, though that was the end of my career with the travellers, perhaps it fed my later love of travel.

My own duel with death began when I was almost five. My dearest brother and playmate (Kevin Patrick) was accidentally killed while harvesting the hay. Many people were there when a sudden downpour sent the men running for cover. My eleven-year-old brother took shelter in the hay and when the rain ceased the men resumed work. One man thought my brother was a pile of hay and dug the pitchfork through his right temple. It was 11th of August 1934, four days before my fifth birthday. My father was in town and my mother, who was busy preparing a festive dinner for the men at the end of the day, told me to go out and play. Running out to find K.P. at the garden gate, I met a neighbour carrying my brother in his outstretched arms. I started to cry and scream and somebody whipped me up in their arms and carried me to my bed. Through the window I could see men's heads: they must have been trying to resuscitate him. I was taken to a neighbour's house that I might calm down, but nothing would console me. Later that day my father came to take me home. I felt comforted in my father's arms. Still in his arms I was taken to say goodbye to my beloved brother, who was laid out on my parents' bed. My mother had made a beautiful pale blue habit and a neighbour wove a crown of white roses for his head which symbolised love and purity. I was desolate. I wanted to lie down beside him and to go to heaven with him. The next day I was allowed to watch the funeral coach with four white horses take my brother away. I knew I could never play with him again.

Today when I hear people say that children will get over things I disagree, because to lose loved ones is like receiving a deep wound in the heart. Such wounds may heal but they leave a scar. My memory has held every detail of that first great loss in my life. Everyone needs to belong, everyone needs to love and be loved, especially children who, in their innocence, claim immediacy and nearness to everything.

After my brother's death I grew very reclusive. In summer I had a favourite hiding place between two double ditches where I played at being a hermit. It was here I began to realise the enormous importance of silence if one wishes to commune with God (the loving essence of life). And it was here I read my first great novel, the Old Testament, at the age of eight. This book has remained in my memory as the best love story of all time, full of drama, prophets and magic. It took me down seemingly familiar paths, especially wandering in the desert for forty years, and Moses' frustration with the people of Israel when they complained of thirst. Moses struck the rock twice and was instantly rebuked by Yahveh for his lack of faith. I imagined I was one of those with little faith.

God said: because you struck the rock twice you will not reach the Promised Land, the land flowing with milk and honey. Aaron your brother will lead My people. Poor Moses died in exile after a life of great virtue and leadership and very little gratitude from the Children of Israel but he will live on as God's mouthpiece, having received the Ten Commandments from Yahveh and delivering them to the people. They are still our code of ethics, but how many of us can remember them?

In Ireland the Old Testament was not recommended reading, but the New Testament was obligatory and when my mother was sold the former instead of the latter it must have been the finger of Fate. That first book left an imprint on me which imparted a complete picture of life, God's forgiveness and His immense love for every one of us, whatever our colour or creed.

CHAPTER 2

INITIATION INTO HEALING

A Sensitive Plant in a garden grew,
And the young winds fed it with silver dew,
And it opened its fan-like leaves to the light,
And closed them beneath the kisses of night.

And the Spring arose on the garden fair,
Like the Spirit of Love felt everywhere;
And each flower and herb on Earth's dark breast
Rose from the dreams of its wintry rest. – Shelley

My father used to say: 'Do not visit anybody with one arm as long as the other.' By which he meant not to go empty-handed, but always take some small gift to your friend or host. This was my initiation into the lavishness and love that was an aspect of the Irish tradition of generosity and hospitality. For my father it was also a conscious expression of his confidence in life. It is my own chief attitude today: be lavish with love. It's the only treasure which multiplies when shared, the only gift which increases when we give it away. Love freely given connects with the life force in another. It is the necessary ingredient in all healing.

Healing and loving have always been synonymous in my life; a pulse coursing through my veins under the vigilant eye of my father, and all of this matured in silence.

My father was our doctor, our nurse, our naturopath. His home-made cures, his potions taken from Mother Earth, cured us all. The doctor's skills were called upon only in a crisis. I only once remember my father telephoning from our village post office to discuss one or other of our symptoms with the doctor.

We were kindred spirits. He was my inspiration and I was his disciple, apprenticed to him in healing though not in farming. He protected me and nurtured my reading and intellectual leanings so that at four years old I could read fluently. Other children were expected to help in one way or another, but no one had the right to disturb me in my reading or writing. I loved reading. I sat on the kitchen table and read aloud to anyone who would listen. I had a strong curiosity and my constant questioning often irritated my mother.

I was never interested in and never played with dolls. I used to lie on the grass in the fields and look at the clouds and imagine God the Father with His big white flowing beard. At other times there would be angels with trumpets announcing the end of the world or horses and riders galloping at fantastic speed and scattering the stars in all directions. Side by side with these spiritual flights of fancy my thoughts would tumble to earth to the wild daisies spread out like a sheet at my feet, then I would long for a pair of black leather shoes with shining buckles to dance a hornpipe on those daisies.

My mother said, 'If you want dancing shoes you have to wish on the stars.' I could not wait for nightfall to fix my eyes on the brightest star and recite my wish:

Star light, star bright
The first star I've seen tonight
I wish I may
I wish I might
Have the wish I wish tonight.

Following this ritual I got my trip to town with my father, who not only bought me my shoes but a beautiful dress as well. My mother also received something special, I remember. On this occasion it was a hat.

The main reading in our house was the *Irish Independent*, the *Messenger of the Sacred Heart* and the *Far East* printed on distinctive light green paper and published by the Maynooth Missions to China. The *Ireland's Own* was a great favourite. I wrote little stories for this magazine (they were never published). I especially enjoyed poetry and fairy tales. We were sent books from my aunt in New York: *Peter Grimes*, *Cinderella*, and the Irish stories of fairies and goblins. Yet I hated school. I was so involved in all that was going on in my father's world and I was learning all the time. I remember vividly how my father used to coax me: sometimes he would place on a big stone a small coin, perhaps a threepenny piece engraved with a rabbit, and tell me that the fairies had left it. If the coin was there I would go off happily. If not, there were tears.

Eventually I adapted to school, where my favourite subjects were reading, writing, religion and needlework. I received at least two first-class prizes for Christian doctrine, which gave my parents great pleasure.

One of my dreams was of finding a potent remedy to heal all mankind. In Ireland, and elsewhere, remedies and cures were handed down from generation to generation. They were often given or exchanged. Prayers and special words (sometimes written down on pieces of paper) went with the remedies. There is a legend that Joseph's donkey sprained his ankle on the flight into Egypt with Mary and the Christ child on his back. Joseph knelt down and put his hands on the donkey's hoof and it was immediately made better. Joseph was the protector of the Holy Family and his name is frequently invoked in healing.

My father had been given St Joseph's cure, and prayer, for sprains and he in turn gave it to me the night before I entered the convent. I lost the piece of paper with the prayer on it, or had to give it up with my other effects when I became a novice – but the cure works nonetheless! My father must have been given it by his mother. Here is a list of the simple remedies I learned at my father's knee:

Warts: Warts disappear when pricked gently with a straight pin. The pin should then be dropped into the hollow stone usually found in cemeteries or sacred sites containing water and called a Blessed Well.

At the age of nine I carried out the instructions of my grandmother. Next morning, I thought nothing of it when the warts had disappeared from both my hands.

Castor oil: This was applied to wounds after cleansing with a dilution of hydrogen peroxide. Often sloughing or weeping wounds would heal up in a week to nine days, leaving not a single scar. When I was burned from a hot pot at my grandmother's house this was the remedy I was given. It left no mark.

Poultices: Heated carbolic soap and sugar solution was applied to gauze, laid over a swelling or joint, then covered with lint and bandage. A few applications saw the end of the problem. Bread poultices applied in a similar way are also effective.

Iodine was used for cuts, painful joints and dog bites. This cure was given to me when I was bitten by a greyhound.

Witch hazel and rose-water was the remedy for bruising and for cleaning the face. For bruising we were also taught to use our saliva and massage the spot as first aid.

For colds and chills – a tiny pinch of fresh ginger in hot milk with a teaspoonful of brandy. Another procedure my father used was camphorated oil on warmed brown paper applied over the chest and back before bedtime and kept in place with a vest all night.

The syrup of figs from the chemist or senna pods we used are still widely employed as a cure for constipation in other cultures.

Sulphur and treacle mixed together was especially good for skin problems and acne. It was also taken as a tonic for the blood.

Aspirin, which is derived from the willow tree, was for colds and fevers.

Cod-liver oil and malt extract we were given as a tonic.

Mumps, measles, whooping cough were treated by bed rest, isolation, and cold compresses, if fever or headaches persisted. We were given a light diet, with plenty of liquids, jelly, custard, rice pudding and soups. When we recovered we got a dose of castor oil with a squeeze of lemon. A teaspoonful of olive oil between three squeezes of lime or lemon first thing in the morning on a fasting stomach is a remedy I rediscovered for stomach ulcers when I trained as a nurse in the Mater Misericordiae Hospital in Dublin in 1950.

Our curate, Father Egan, gave my father a cure for ringworm: it was an ointment, made up to a special recipe and contained in little white ceramic jars. Ringworm is a fungus occasionally found in cattle and can be contagious.

At the age of twelve, in November 1941, I developed rheumatic fever. I was fasting and had cycled in the rain to a special Mass, then cycled that afternoon to another town to buy a dress for my godchild's first birthday. I was tired and couldn't eat when I returned home. In the night I developed a fever. I was taken over to our barn across the way for nursing. I was unable to move from pains in my joints and had a huge temperature and headache. I could only swallow from a bottle. On Sunday my father came to attend to me and found I had the death rattle in my throat. He said he was going to send for the doctor and the priest. I signalled I did not want them. My father went to his bedroom, fell on his knees and implored Our Lady of Perpetual Succour to save me. He returned to find me sitting up and asking for a drink of water: his prayers had been answered. From that point on my convalescence started. I missed a lot of school and read many novels which I stole from my father's bookcase.

The barn had an interesting history. It was a big, single-storey room with a fireplace and a double bed that could fold up like a wardrobe. In Ireland this was called a press bed. Shortly after building the barn, my grandfather fell ill. When the priest came to see him he said, 'You have fallen ill because you have built this house out of line and on the old people's path. You must put it in line with the dwelling house.' When this was done my grandfather got up from his bed and was immediately full of health. The room was kept for special occasions or when someone was ill and needed quiet and peace. My memory of it is as a healing place and, as I understand it, all healing is linked to a spiritual awareness. This barn standing alone harnessing every spiritual, physical and mental energy was like a holy refuge and it was close to the path of the spirits.

In retrospect I see the priest as a sort of Feng Shui expert, sensitive to spiritual energies. In our lives and our sicknesses we need people around us who are compassionate and can alleviate our pain – pain which can invade us at many levels. Priests, carers, nurses, practitioners, doctors all have their place, but they must look after themselves too. Prolonged periods of overwork can consume their energies and endanger their own health – in taking care of others they should never forget the importance of prayer. Those of us who practise as professionals or otherwise share in a Divine process and, like a great work of art, the results can uplift us to the very gates of Heaven.

At that time in Ireland turning the soul to God in prayer was a common practice. The Morning Offering was said on rising. At midday and at six in the evening the Angelus bell rang out, as depicted by Millet in his painting, *The Angelus*. Every child was taught to say the Prayer to their Guardian Angel at bedtime:

> O Angel of God
> My guardian dear
> To whom God's love commits me here
> Ever this night be at my side
> To light and guard
> To rule and guide. Amen.

CHAPTER 3

VOCATION TO A FRENCH ORDER AND TRAINING AS A NURSE

Before I formed you in the womb, I knew you:
Before you came to birth I consecrated you.
I have appointed you as prophet to the nations . . .
So now brace yourself for action. Stand up and tell them all
  I command you.
They will fight against you but shall not overcome you, for
  I am with you to deliver you. – Jeremiah 1: 4–5, 17–19

At the age of sixteen, the year the Second World War came to an end, I visited a convent with a girl whose close friend had recently joined. This convent was in Dublin, but the order of nuns was started in France around 1839 by a young French woman from Brittany, who wanted to devote her life to the care of the aged, the sick and infirm of all denominations. Today the order has spread over five continents and the foundress has been declared Blessed by our Holy Father the Pope.

The life of these nuns and their unselfish devotion struck a chord in my own soul. I wanted to learn, to further my education, and I wanted complete freedom from worldly cares, so as to love God in His poor. My early years had filled my mind and imagination with a desire to serve. Without a doubt I heard the call and my mind was made up very quickly.

References were taken up and I entered the convent as a postulant six months later. A film called *The Song of Bernadette* was showing in Dublin at that time, I went to see it and was extremely moved by the little French girl who saw the Blessed Virgin Mary at Lourdes eighteen times from the 11th of February to the 16th of July 1858. I was overcome by Bernadette's humility and her reply when asked, who was God? 'God is Love,' she said with a pure, convincing voice. I was pleased that I too was going to learn to love God in a French order! The example of St Bernadette confirmed my resolution.

My father took me to the train. The night before, he had given me the special prayer to St Joseph, with a cure for sprains. On the way we were silent; no words could have expressed our heartbreak. Arriving at Dromod railway station my father took me in his arms, kissed me and said, 'If you don't like it, please don't stay – come home.' I waved goodbye until the train gathered speed and he was lost to view. When I had told my parents about my decision to join the convent they were very happy and no doubt proud – and perhaps expected me home after the weekend, but I never returned. I sat on the train for Dublin, lost in reverie; the green fields were speeding past and, though I knew I'd miss my parents, my thoughts were full of God and my new life.

In Dublin, I took a taxi to the convent in Kilmainham and was received with open arms by the Superior and Sister Julienne, who had charge of the postulant's first steps and training for the apostolate. This was a kind of six-month probation period when either side could change their minds.

I was shown to my bed in the large attic dormitory. I remember I was pleased I had a corner one. My civilian clothes were taken away and I donned my first religious habit. Immediately I felt at home in it – a frilly bonnet, dark camisole, skirt, black shoes and stockings, and a short cape over the shoulders.

The mattress was of straw in imitation of Christ in the manger. The pallet had a split opening: once a week we had to push our hands through this and toss the straw. The bed was made up with white sheets. A locker by the side held a jug, basin, soap on a round saucer, and the lower shelf held a 'po', or chamber-pot, and towel. Bell for rising was rung at 5.30 a.m. At the sound, we all 'raised our hearts to God', jumped out of bed, washed in cold water, dressed, emptied slops into a bucket placed on a mat in the middle of the dormitory and hurried to the oratory for meditation. This was followed by Holy Mass and Communion. Thus our spiritual needs were seen to at the beginning of the day. Breakfast followed at 8 a.m.: coffee, bread and butter, with jam or fruit on feast days. The food, in those post-war days, was adequate but plain.

Then we went to our designated service to help with the old people's breakfast, and later to aid the more invalid amongst them, to bathe and dress. To some they would have been the dregs of society but we were taught to treat prince and pauper alike. Our days were made up of prayer, study and work serving the poor. The convent and the main building formed part of a complex which also housed the elderly people, some of whom enjoyed helping the sisters in the running of the house and garden.

The rules were strict but for postulants the most difficult was the observance of silence, both in word and in action. Total discretion was expected and we were not allowed to enquire into each other's backgrounds. We knew we were all of 'good seed' (i.e. respectable families) – that was one of the requirements of entry. We had to be physically, mentally and spiritually well adjusted. Our group, the Sainte Marie, were particularly noted for their religious fervour, but our happiness was important – no sad-faced saints were allowed. One postulant was so funny at making silly faces that she used to send us into ripples of suppressed laughter. Then, on hearing footsteps, we would have to regain our composure quickly. She of course kept a dead serious face which was beyond suspicion!

Nowadays the discipline might be regarded as harsh, but it has stood me in good stead throughout my life. The convent training as a whole undoubtedly enabled me to move freely among all sorts and conditions of people. I do realise, though, that I am talking about an age which had a very different attitude towards the upbringing of young people. Humility and obedience were to be our shield and our breastplate. Silence and discretion were instilled into us. No radios, no telephones, no newspapers – nothing – distracted us from the noble calling we had embraced with such ardour. Up to the present day I still love my silence and my need for it is as great as my need for books or sunshine. In silence we possess our souls.

But we had our recreational times, our studies and many hours of sheer happiness and laughter – love has to be directed and must come from a spiritual source. On *our* journey the source of love was Christ, who favoured the weak and the pure of heart. We were students of His love.

> When you can say with entire truth and with a whole heart: Lord God, lead me wherever thou desirest, then and only then do you deliver yourself from servitude and become really free. (*Thoughts of the Wise*)

As I look back now I see the blessings which were scattered on our lives; heroic deeds were being done without a second thought. It could only have been possible through the gift of Faith and the unquestioning acceptance of my vocation to follow Christ wherever He led me, or to be carried by Him if I faltered *en route*. Serving Christ gives tremendous peace and confidence. It allows one to throw off ambition and the quest for worldly goods, and it frees the soul.

We were all in love with Christ, and expressed this through service to His suffering old people, whose families could no longer cope. We owned nothing and wanted for nothing. Everything we had was dependent on the generosity of our many benefactors, who held the work in veneration.

After six months, the postulants were admitted to the noviciate. Here the real work began of 'putting on the new woman'. Entering the religious life meant no holidays and never returning home. Personal belongings were not allowed, letters to parents were censored, visits from family discouraged.

We studied theology, the French language and many other subjects that related to our lives as religious. As an order dedicated to Christ, we followed the rule of St Augustine. Born in Thagaste, North Africa in AD 354 of a pagan father and Christian mother, Augustine was a brilliant young man whose early life was wild and unsettled: he loved beautiful women. Later, he was converted to Christianity by the prayers of his mother (St Monica) and was baptised in AD 387. He returned to Africa where he lived an ascetic life and eventually became Bishop of Hippo. His writings have been extremely influential, particularly to religious communities, because they present a theology and spirituality which are gentle and adaptable. When he found Christ all his utterances were of Love.

Study, prayer, penance and household duties filled our days, from our rising at 5.30 a.m. until the day ended at 9.30 p.m. After we had said our office, 'Great Silence' was announced by the sound of the bell and we had to be in bed. I loved the peace and stillness of the night when the spirit could go where it pleased. In the convent there were no mirrors to help us dress, and we were forbidden to gaze at ourselves in glass doors – surprisingly difficult for a young woman in love with her calling!

Often I had to confess my vanity on this point and do the prescribed penance.

Once a week there was a chapter of faults. Each novice took her place, kneeling in the centre of the oratory, confessing her faults in public and receiving a penance according to the gravity of the fault. Generally the penance was the recitation of a psalm or other prayer but sometimes it was major, and one had to beg for one's bread in the refectory or eat one's dinner in the middle of the floor on a small stool. I had to do this a few times during my eighteen months as a novice, when I had been distracted and caught dreaming. Were dreams always to be my downfall? I felt very humiliated but was comforted by thinking of Christ's humiliations during His passion. Christ said to the rich young man in the Gospel, 'Unless you leave father and mother and all worldly goods you cannot be my disciple.' My great desire was to become the spouse of Christ, not just a disciple, so the exchange seemed a fair one. I was aged nineteen years and four months when I pronounced my first temporary vows on 8th of December 1948. To belong at last to a Divine Spouse was my dearest wish. We were all dressed in bridal robes and veils with crowns of white roses on our heads. Prostrate before the altar, I felt it was a solemn moment: our hearts were pounding and filled with love for Christ while we pronounced our vows of poverty, chastity, obedience and hospitality.

My mother and father were there. I had not seen them since I entered. They were so happy and moved to tears by the ceremony. We joined our families for a festive lunch and at last met our colleagues' parents. Our mutual happiness was brimming over, with undercurrents of sadness at having to say goodbye to parents. I did not realise then that I would never see my father again and my mother only once, when I left the convent in 1965. Happily the future is hidden from us.

Preparation for this big occasion was a ten-day retreat in complete silence. The night before our profession of vows our hair was shorn. This symbolised casting off all worldly things as we put on the close-fitting white headdress and the black habit which I loved. A few months later I was sent to study nursing in the Mater Misericordiae Hospital in Dublin run by the Sisters of Mercy. I was overjoyed by this since my innate curiosity about healing found new scope in my medical studies while I could still hold on to the natural ways which my father had taught me. I was one of the first group of our order to take this medical training; we were six. Our visionary Mother Provincial had foreseen the need for trained nurses to provide better care for the aged in our houses around the world. As nurses, we had to wear white habits over which we fitted our black cloaks when we were off-duty – the combination was lovely!

My first assignment was to a medical ward called St Laurence, where quite a number of young men were suffering from TB. I was hopelessly shy and when a young man confined to complete bed rest at the end of the ward by the window asked me for a urinal, it took me time and a lot of blushes to bring the much-needed object to his bedside. I, who had run away from the world, was plunged back into a new world of sickness and pain. Often I had to assist the patients to die – having no idea that my whole life was to become a duel with that ravager of life.

I became very friendly with that lovely patient confined to bed and we had wonderful exchanges of thought on books, poetry and the things of God. He had lost his father suddenly when he was in college. He had wanted to be a farmer before he was struck down by tuberculosis. I nursed him and nurtured him. He was my ideal of the perfect man: fatalistic, not complaining, but seeing the best in everything and living each day as it came. He subsequently wrote me wonderful letters.

On the whole I loved the time passed in study and training. I learned fast and my natural diagnostic skills, inherited from my father and nurtured by him, were often in demand by the young housemen-doctors who came to me for ward experience.

After three years I was to sit my finals in Trinity College Dublin with special permission from the Pope to attend a Protestant university. This seemed a wonderful place to me, peaceful yet full of energy. After I passed I went back to the hospital to bid farewell to the nuns who had trained me and of course to certain patients! On the back stairs I met an anaesthetist with whom I had worked. To my astonishment, he begged me to leave the convent and marry him. He was deadly serious – I ran for my life. In retrospect I see it as a final invitation from the world to return to its fold. How innocent I was, even raw, in worldly wisdom.

Innocence is precious and powerful: not to be confused with ignorance, it is a Divine protection against the negative forces of life. We grow wise by stages and often a whole lifetime of experience is necessary to gain wisdom. 'Wisdom is glorious,' said King Solomon, 'and never fadeth away.' It is a pity, though, that our young people lose their innocence so much earlier than they used to. And that it's often the false prophets and vain gossipers who are most often listened to and even idolised (the icons of today).

Back in the convent I missed the hospital life – the familiar faces of nuns and doctors, the changing faces of the many patients. But I was soon able to put my knowledge to good use. One afternoon, my Superior asked me to have a look at our chauffeur, Mr Gannon, who was complaining of a pain in his chest. I examined him, took his blood pressure and pulse rate. I did not like what I found and asked him to go to Casualty. That evening, my Superior called me out of chapel to tell me Mr Gannon was dead: instead of going straight to Casualty, he had returned home to see his wife and children. He told his wife what I had said and gave her his pay packet.

As Mrs Gannon stood on the doorstep, waving goodbye to her husband, his car careered to the side of the road. Her husband had died at the wheel, doing the job he loved. Next day my name hit the headlines – I was the last medical person to have seen him and there was to be an inquest. The post-mortem revealed an enlarged heart, which had gone into failure and was beyond repair. I was glad he had said goodbye to his wife. Now I know the suffering involved in heart surgery, I think no differently.

On the 31st of October 1952, with other sisters from my group, I sailed to France for a further year of religious study. It was so exciting going to France for the first time. The Channel crossing was rough and it was a relief to mount the train which took us to our Mother House. From the carriage windows we saw the countryside robed in its autumnal colours and I was captivated by the mystical beauty of Brittany. The Mother House was a large château set in hundreds of acres of land. Its enormous flagstoned corridors held a great temptation to make a noise, which of course we could not do. This year was going to be a testing one on all levels. Though I had learned French by now so could converse easily, the food was different for a start. The cider at mealtimes completely upset me, but when I sought permission to drink water instead, I was refused and told 'not to be seeking attention'. About a month later, getting out of bed at 5.30 a.m., I collapsed. I do not remember being carried to the infirmary – my temperature was very high and I had a lot of abdominal pain caused by too much acidity in the cider. I remember the early morning cooing of the wood pigeons and the birdsong outside the infirmary window. It must have been springtime. After blood tests and bed rest, I resumed normal life but my diet had changed: cider was forbidden and weekly injections were given, including vitamin B12 and intravenous injections of calcium.

On the 15th of October 1953, the feast day of the Great Theresa of Avila, I once again made my solemn vows of poverty, chastity, obedience and hospitality. The vow of hospitality was peculiar to our order and has remained very important to me. The vow of chastity somehow never posed a problem for me. I simply had a wonderful feeling of belonging to God for ever. We were a very large group from the four corners of the world; as we waited for our 'obedience', our first assignment as fully fledged nuns, I wondered, by now with acceptance, about my destination. Would it be a far-flung mission? Alas, I was sent back to Dublin Noviciate as counsellor and nurse to the community. I was also in charge of the chapel, the door, the phone and visitors – like the PR of the House. The Noviciate was called The Hermitage and as a novice I had loved its peace and silence. Nevertheless, a tiny part of me had hoped to be sent abroad.

As a young nun, I knew things would be very different, responsibilities heavy at times. There were many challenges, but some of the challenges came, not from the outside world but from within the religious community; one particular incident comes to mind. Every year we renewed our vows on the 8th of December, the feast of Mary Immaculate, a ceremony preceded by ten days in retreat. One evening after the lecture, I went to the priest's quarters to put coal on the fire and draw the curtains. I was on my knees before the fire when Father came in. I rose and made for the door but the priest barred it and tried to embrace me. I pushed him away and left. My heart was racing. I had never expected the advances of a priest – especially a retreat master!

Immediately I made up my mind: I would not tell a soul, I would not divulge the incident lest he be sent away or get a bad reputation with his bishop. The next year, on a different retreat, another priest did the same thing. Again, I kept silent. Years later another priest in France told me of his attraction to me; from all three instances I learned that priests are men and men are human, and that silence is golden.

One morning a priest requested to say Mass. He signed his name and I recognised it as that of a priest from home. Many years before he had fainted while celebrating Sunday Mass in our local church in Ireland. I mentioned this to the novice mistress, who begged me not to leave her alone with him. Luckily I did not, because he collapsed at almost the same point in the Mass once again. He told me later that he was a mild epileptic and had forgotten to take his medicine. It had not happened for years but that morning he had forgotten to take his tablet. Then, it was my father who had jumped over the altar rails to give him treatment. I was dying to tell him that I had been present and that it had been my father who had helped him but I refrained, because our religious rules asked for silence about our families and it was an exercise in humility not to indulge in self-praise.

CHAPTER 4

FOUR YEARS IN INDIA

Fused with endless night, I came to rest
At the altar of the stars. Alone, amazed, I stared
Upwards with hands clasped and said: 'Sun you have
  removed
Your rays: show now your loveliest, kindliest form
That I may see the Person who dwells in me as in you.'

— Tagore

The child of eight dreaming of China could not have known that revolution and Mao Tse Tung's Red Army would close that country's door to foreigners for decades to come. The nun of twenty-eight had also to amend her dreams; if she couldn't be a missionary in China, she would still be a missionary – somewhere.

At the age of twenty-nine, in 1958, my request to become a missionary was granted by my Head Superior and India was to be my destination – first Bombay and, after two months, Calcutta. I set myself the task of finding out what I could about the country, and Calcutta in particular. The encyclopaedia seemed to call Calcutta a Black Hole! I did not understand the terminology and feared the worst, yet was still very excited about a new adventure.

It was only when preparations for my departure were far

advanced that it was discovered I had not been vaccinated as a child, and in quick succession I received all of them: smallpox, typhoid, yellow fever, cholera. The effects were disastrous; high fever and exhaustion pinned me to my bed for ten days, my life weighed in the balance. (It is now known that vaccinations given indiscriminately can cause death.) The journey was postponed until I was declared fit to travel.

Another young sister was to be my companion as far as Bombay. We were supposed to go by boat, but once again the great wheel of history rolled up against the little wheel of my life: the Suez Canal crisis had flared up two years earlier and as the Canal was still closed we flew to India instead – a great adventure in those days. From the experience of that long, bumpy air trip, it is the image of the Egyptian desert which stays in my mind. My eyes feasted on a vast expanse of purple and brown turning to a rainbow of colour as the sun rose.

I'll never forget my first sight, and first smell, of Bombay. The monsoon was over, it was November, and life felt good. It is the colours that hit you first, then the smell – an acrid fug – next the noise, all the hustle and bustle. Then the poverty: the crowded, dirty streets and the ragged people. In my wildest dreams I had never conjured up an image like that mass of humanity, sprawling on the ground, the poorest, or the sickest of the poor, simply curled up in the filthy gutters.

I had been assigned to help a petite Canadian sister, who was there to start a new home for the aged poor, and we had been loaned a modest house in Bandra which lies on the outskirts of

Bombay, where there were no comforts of any kind. Like campers, we slept on makeshift beds – when the strange nocturnal noises allowed us to sleep. In the clearing of a neglected garden we cooked our meagre ration of vegetables and rice on a little kerosene lamp and we shared the delicious fruits of India.

The smells and the poverty were difficult to contend with. We lived on alms alone, which was possible since the Indian people are spiritually minded and understand the language of love. However, begging for alms to enable our work to continue had to be abandoned when darkness suddenly fell at six o'clock in the evening: we carried no watches. On my first-hand encounter with the streets of Bombay I was constantly shocked by the poverty, the acrid smells, the under-nourished children – the mother with three babies all at the same time tugging at her breasts, extracting the last ounce of her strength. My companion was intrepid in spite of being of slight build. We never had the least fear – our religious habit was our pass to freedom and respect.

The men had the easy jobs like sitting at machines tailoring or working as vendors in the market-place, while the women were coolies, washerwomen or carried bricks on their heads to the builder. It seemed to me that except as a wife, mother or worker, women had no value, were not considered, never had a chance – often they fell on their knees after the smallest kindness, wanting to kiss my feet, crying 'Amma', mother. I felt I should have been on my knees kissing their feet: it makes one feel very humble to witness such humility and resignation.

Christ said in His Sermon on the Mount, 'Blessed are the meek for they shall inherit the earth. Blessed are the poor in spirit for theirs is the kingdom of Heaven.' I cannot forget the woman who had only a handful of rice yet insisted we take half. I was so moved to see such poverty and such generosity. I was reminded of 'the widow's mite', the parable where Christ says that the rich give out of their abundance and the poor out of their love.

The days were too short. Often, returning to Bandra, the sun would surprise us by setting suddenly and leaving us in relative darkness to get home as best we could. After a small supper my companion and I would say office together and retire to bed, where we tried to sleep, amid the ghostly sounds of the night creatures on the prowl. After about three months, my train journey was booked to Calcutta. The Canadian sister and I said goodbye at the railway station. In my naivety I expected the journey to take about twelve hours and had come with just a few bananas. Instead, it took thirty-six – two whole days and a night. Providence looked after me, in the shape of a pious Parsee lady who shared all her bread and rancid butter (difficult for an Irish country girl!) throughout the journey.

At Nagpur, known as the city of oranges, at last I quenched my thirst with some great oranges which I bought on the platform with my last rupees. What a treat, what a luxury those oranges were! Washing facilities on the train were non-existent. Anyone who has travelled in India third-class like the poor will be familiar with carriages that are little better than cattle carts, seats and ground space completely littered with people, chickens and rolled-up parcels of food. To get to the one and only overstretched toilet, passengers had to crawl over bodies. I was dressed all in white, but when I arrived in Calcutta I must have been a sorry sight. Two sisters were waiting for me on the platform. I was home at last.

When I took up my post as nurse and counsellor in the convent I was presented to the community in a formal ceremony in the oratory. The convent was a haven of peace. I was given the ladies' infirmary to look after – about sixty old ladies, some confined to bed, but others ambulant and able to help in the running of the place. The work was strenuous, the climate arduous, but youth and faith give their own strength and all went well for a time. From December to February the days were dry and pleasant, but when the monsoon came the heat and humidity were relentless. There was no point in drying after a shower. The simplest act became a trial of strength.

Another nun was working in Calcutta while I was there: Mother Teresa, who had stayed briefly in our convent several years before, when she was laying down the foundations for what would become her Sisters of Charity. She was then unknown to the world, but her work of rescuing poor people from the streets of Calcutta was already attracting attention among her fellow religious. She was in her early fifties then – but to me she seemed ancient! Already she walked with the stoop the world would come to know so well from all those hours bent over in Calcutta's streets. Mother Teresa lived in her own convent at this time and devoted all her time to the dying. She was out on the streets at dawn with her little ambulance, scanning the gutters. Leaves and moving matter were a signal to her and she would clear the debris with her bare hands to find the human mass underneath. One incident created great public interest at the time. One morning she pulled out a woman in a terrible condition – maggots had already begun to eat her flesh, yet she was still conscious, murmuring prayers to God to rescue her. Mother Teresa took the woman in her arms, wrapped her in a clean sheet and did what she did with all of the poor she rescued: she transported the woman back to her hospice, bathed her and wrapped her in a clean, white sari. The woman whispered, 'I was praying to God I wouldn't die in the gutter.' She died moments later.

I was inspired by Mother Teresa's courage. When I visited her hospice I was struck by an amazing aura of light which I perceived as a spiritual presence, even though the hospice was just one huge room with little natural light. It was filled to capacity with dying people on camp-beds, assisted by the Sisters of Charity. I know Mother Teresa did excellent work, but she, and others before her, ignored the very real needs of the mothers and children. This, to me, was the most pertinent subject which was not being addressed by any of them. It seemed clear that mothers and babies were experiencing unimaginable suffering and I witnessed this at first hand. It made me think about how Christ took the child and set him in the midst of his disciples and said, 'Anyone who welcomes one of these little children in my name welcomes me, and anyone who welcomes me, welcomes not me, but the One who sent me.'

As I was the only fully qualified nurse in my community, my Superior often asked me to help with medical problems. I frequently did the work of a doctor, stitching after accidents and undertaking other medical interventions. I remember a woman who was blue in the face and struggling for life after having swallowed a chicken bone. I put my hand down her throat and worked to dislodge it, restoring her breathing to normal.

My greatest shock was when I was asked to help with a young pregnant mother who was overdue and in difficulties. I was able to advise her medically but urged her to see a doctor because her condition was serious. I explained I was not a midwife and did not have the knowledge. Three days later I learned from her young husband that she had died with the baby still in her uterus. This tragedy affected us all deeply as her husband was known to us and at Mass every morning assisted our chaplain and the community with great fervour. The drama and grief of this young husband raised serious doubts in my mind. I asked myself many questions about my own vocation and the work of our order, which was strictly dedicated to the care of the elderly regardless of their religion. Mother Teresa was also concerned with the aged. What value do we put on human life, on human suffering? It seemed that women and babies were being left to perish.

All we need is Love but love without knowledge falls short. A dream of some day practising midwifery and teaching my skills began to take shape. Another dream was added to my previous ones.

Young mothers were dying because they had no one to educate or guide them. Contraception was unheard of, doctors were scarce and medical care was harnessed to looking after 'burned' (suttee) cases, which took their toll of hospitals and staff. These were people who had tried to take their own lives by setting themselves alight; women in particular sought this desperate escape from their terrible existence or were even set on fire by members of their own families. There were beds of burned patients whose sloughing wounds were indescribable – not to mention odours. Their suffering was appalling.

Doctors were overworked, nurses never knew holidays. When was there time to teach the simplest principles of antenatal care? The hospitals were overcrowded and chaotic. Families who brought food for their sick unwittingly added more stress to the already hard-pressed nursing team – but these were the customs, and the family of each patient believed that their presence would help to heal the sick family member. Many of the diseases were caused by neglect and lack of hygiene. I saw the problems clearly, but my commitment had already been made to care for the aged, poor and dying and I was obedient to my order.

The mental strain of the work and the climate began to affect my own health. After a short period in the infirmary, with a tubercular lesion on my lung, I got my obedience to our home in Secunderabad in Andhra Pradesh. Once again I filled the post of counsellor and had charge of a huge infirmary of male patients with very little help. Poor children, ragged and hungry, came to the gate and to our dining room in search of a handful of rice. I often got into trouble for feeding the children and encouraging the beggars. I saw these people as Children of God – how could I not give them something to eat? I could hear my father saying, if a poor person comes to the door never turn them away. A lovely and holy little man used to help me: his name was Gabriel, his heart was bigger than the world, and his requests for the little ones I could not resist.

My faith was being tested as I was torn between my duty towards the aged poor served by my own community and the children and the mothers I saw all around me. The words of a French poet Théodore Monet (written at the age of seven) came to mind and gave me strength:

> Que ma Foi soit mon toit
> et la Bonté mon rez-de-chaussée.

> (Let my Faith be my rooftop
> and Goodness my ground floor.)

When I think about my life I see it as one of learning through trials and tribulations, with the odd patch of blue sky and clear water. The year of 1962 brought tragedy and transformation. In August I received word that my father was very ill. On the night of the 26th, we prayed that he might be cured. I remember going to bed at 9 p.m. I was on call if anybody needed help in the night. It was very hot as I pulled the mosquito net around me and settled beneath the sheets.

At once I caught sight of a figure, parting the curtain which surrounded the bed and approaching. I thought I was seeing Christ – he was wearing a white robe with a sash. He put both his hands to my face and kissed me – exactly as my father used to do. I was spellbound. I could not speak. I wanted to ask for my father's cure. The apparition put his hands to my face again, kissed me and left through the same point in the curtain as he had entered. I got up, looked at the clock and found it was only 9.10 p.m. All this had happened in ten minutes. My soul was exalted. I did not return to bed but prayed and enjoyed the gift I had received. Next morning, I told my charges that maybe our prayers had been answered, that my father had been cured.

On my return from the local hospital late that morning, my Superior called me to her office. A telegram had come saying that my father had died at 3 p.m. with my name on his lips, thanking God that I was looking after God's poor in India: 3 p.m. in Ireland would have been 9 p.m. in India. So it was my father, himself, who paid me that unique visit on the previous night! I never shed a tear – I knew he was with God – my soul felt an incredible peace. The vision I had had of him the previous night stayed with me and consoles me even to the present day.

Again, due to overwork, my health problems returned. This time I could not eat or drink anything. I was hospitalised for a week in Hyderabad General Hospital, the only European in a huge ward. The matron visited me every day and showed me great kindness. She never came without bringing me something: I remember the passion fruit and how I loved their colour and crinkled texture. X-rays revealed severe inflammation throughout the alimentary tract and cancer of the large intestine. The sad verdict was brought to me by the matron, that I would have to return to Europe for treatment, but with the warning that I must never be operated upon. (This was to be proven beyond doubt years later.)

The news of my condition and that I had to leave India was horrible – I would have preferred death. By this time I no longer noticed the smell of India and felt completely at home there. My ideal was to live and die in India and perhaps have my remains fed to the hungry birds from one of those high towers. Once I observed a funny incident when a messenger delivering a large sack of meat was suddenly swooped upon by a vulture and his parcel of meat disappeared into the air. I'm sure the vulture's hungry family had a feast. I would have been happy to end as such a meal and give the birds a treat.

I had two dreams about this time. In one I saw the Virgin Mary in the heavens with the Christ Child held between her outstretched hands. She was blessing the world with the Child. The second dream was a huge cross in the skies, illuminated with stars. My interpretation of the first dream was that mothers and children were to be my first concern. The second dream showed me that I was signed with the cross and that life would not be easy. These two dreams helped me to become reconciled with my departure from India. I hoped and prayed that somehow my longing to work with mothers and children would be realised in living or in dying.

I knew that to fulfil my vocation I had to learn midwifery, though how it would come about I could not foresee. I returned to Europe by jet, which was unusual in 1962, and I remember lying across several seats feeling extremely unwell. My destination was France, the beautiful cathedral town of Autun in Burgundy. I had spent four years in India and was now seriously ill . . .

CHAPTER 5

LEAVING THE CONVENT

The regeneration of humanity can only be accomplished
if we take care of our children, even before they are
born, which means we must take care of the pregnant
mother. – Omraam Mikhael Aivanhov

If we have a goal in life, work becomes like mountaineering. We have a view of the role we want to play: a vision of becoming a complete person, contributing both as an individual and as one of humankind. One stands at the foot of the mountain and the climb seems easy, but after the first few hours it becomes difficult, you get tired, you rest, then the path clears, only to get difficult again before the summit – but what joy and what ecstasy on reaching the top where the canopy of Heaven is all-embracing . . .

At thirty-three years of age, in a convent in Autun, France, I thought I had reached the limit of my endurance and that it would be the perfect age to die. My health was declining. I now weighed six stone and, according to one of the girls whom I had trained, my colour was yellowish green. Thank God for the absence of mirrors – otherwise I might have worried! I asked no questions about my condition, I was longing to die and I thought I could see the summit. To my mind, suffering with cancer was the fine-tuning needed for the last lap of the journey. I was not fearful: on the contrary I was full of joy to be going home to God at such a young age.

In spite of my serious health problems I was given charge of the ladies' infirmary and *pharmacie* with four young girls who gave us their youth and their beauty at weekends and during the summer holidays, helping to care for the sick and learning how to do it professionally. For the first time since my final vows, I did not hold the post of counsellor, but had great joy teaching those eager young girls to fulfil their dreams: they all became qualified nurses except Marie-France who came to England to study midwifery. On the eve of her final exam she left to marry an Englishman, and she had also fallen in love with England.

My Superior, whom we called Bonne Mère, was also a trained nurse and very sympathetic. Short, slim and in her early forties – with a beautiful smile – she allowed me a long siesta in the afternoon and to go earlier to bed and later to rise than normal; evidently work must have been the antidote which my superiors imagined might cure me. Medically it seemed I was past treatment but a vegetarian diet was recommended with a syrup which greatly alleviated the pain of swallowing. Whether I ate or fasted I experienced the same type of pain and often I was rolling on the floor in agony. However, the compassion of the Bonne Mère indicated genuine love and she often consulted with Dr Cusson.

*

For all the rigours of life, I loved this house. It was a happy place. The Superior had a free spirit – she understood the needs of her community. She was good to the aged poor and often spoiled them. The food was simple, country fare, though excellent, but I dared not partake of it – my diet was a plain bland one of steamed vegetables and milk puddings.

There were certain authors we were not allowed to read without our Superior's permission, such as the great mystics, St Theresa of Avila and St John of the Cross. Born in sixteenth-century Spain, Theresa was only thirteen years of age when her mother died. In November 1536 she entered the Carmelite Convent of the Incarnation but had to leave after two years due to ill health and return to her family. In 1561 she founded the first convent of the reformed Carmelites with St John of the Cross, who was her confessor and superb spiritual director. I was longing to read their books and Bonne Mère gave me permission. Both were great sources of inspiration and I am sure that they did much for me in my spiritual search and in my recovery. They are still among my favourites and I often dip into them for inspiration. All went well, until the appointment of the new Assistant Bonne Mère. She was Spanish, had a wonderful singing voice but, alas! was scornful of what she saw as 'special privileges'. This was to bring the much-loved Bonne Mère and the whole house into great disarray.

In the Summer of 1963 our Bonne Mère was returning from her annual retreat for Superiors, and the sisters and old people were preparing a little feast for her homecoming. I went to the kitchen to make a special cake for the occasion with Sister Micheline, who had enlisted my help. As I stooped down to take a cake tin from a lower shelf, my back went. A searing pain shot through me, I was unable to move and had to be carried to the infirmary. There I had to lie absolutely flat for a week. Dr Cusson administered a shot of pethidine. 'If you want to recover, you cannot hope to do it and remain in the convent,' he told me, but I ignored these wise words.

Our lovely Superior arrived back to general celebrations. I was comforted by the fact that Sister Micheline had finished the cake, which had been all ready to go into its tin. As I was confined to bed I had a private visit from Bonne Mère.

For six months I got around almost completely bent in two, despite prescribed medicines. My lower spine was wedged and nothing gave me respite. One day Bonne Mère called me to her office and told me about a bone-setter in Autun. She gave me a very nice sister, Anne-Marie, to accompany me to this great healer. He pulled and stretched me, and then, with a gadget that looked like an electric iron, ironed out my back and gave me a couple of painkillers. I returned to the convent erect and standing six feet tall in the joy of my new-found freedom. From that moment my health slowly began to improve and to this day I've had no recurrence of that back pain.

The following year, again during the Bonne Mère's retreat, a visit from the Mother Provincial's Assistant was suddenly announced. The object of this visit was a mystery to me at the time, but to my amazement I was asked to go to Algiers, where

I was told I was urgently needed. Although I was shocked, again I did not ask any questions (we had no right to question obedience) but my health was still not good, I had not been given the all-clear from the cancer. This same Superior accompanied me to Marseilles. I was left there, awaiting another sister as companion to Algiers. So what was all the hurry about? I thought. The move could have waited until the return of the Bonne Mère – I had not been able to thank her for all her guidance, healing and love.

About two days after my arrival in Marseilles, in chapel during Mass I heard familiar footsteps. I raised my head and could not believe my eyes: it was none other than the young sixteen-year-old girl Marie-France, one of my pupils from Autun, in her green and black pleated tartan skirt. At the end of Mass, she and her mother were waiting in the corridor. As I passed them on my way to help with the breakfast, I innocently asked what had brought them to Marseilles. Marie-France embraced me and gave me a folded note, saying, 'Now our mission is accomplished.' The note, which was not even in an envelope, was from the Bonne Mère. In it, she told me that when she returned from her retreat, she found the whole community in schism. It had been reported that Bonne Mère, myself and a few others had formed a forbidden league of friendship and were showing too much kindness to an old couple whose only son had committed suicide. When Bonne Mère was accused, she left the convent and, in spite of coaxing and other means, could not be persuaded to return. This was a huge blow to the Major Superiors (in charge of a group of communities of the same order), who up to this point had never found fault with her administration. The accusations were unjustified. Dumbfounded, I had to re-read the note three times to grasp its meaning. I then tore it into pieces and put it down the lavatory. My mind was stunned by the treachery which maligned a great Superior and I felt an enormous sadness invade my whole being.

When finally I flew to Algiers in the company of the Mother Provincial, I had a lot to think about. On arrival I was given charge of the men's infirmary with little or no help. It was very dirty and I knew my health would suffer. A couple of months later, remembering Dr Cusson's advice, I sat in my tiny room and wrote to Pope Paul VI, asking permission to leave the congregation on grounds of ill health, with the intention of studying midwifery and later returning to the missions to care for mothers and babies – if it were God's will. The Pope received my letter and granted permission. My official document allowing me to leave was dated the 5th of August 1965: I would be thirty-six years of age on the 15th. Incidentally, the only person we could write to without censorship was the Pope. I am sure I was the very first to take that literally. How I did it, to this day I cannot say – it must have been in the Divine Plan.

However, my years in the convent were not wasted. A great Superior had shown me the way. I had learned above all to love and trust God as a little child – no amount of petty jealousy can undermine or weaken that love, which undoubtedly strengthened my decision to leave the convent, save my health and fulfil my dream of becoming a midwife. I returned briefly to France, where the Superior tried to dissuade me, but no one ever mentioned the fact that Bonne Mère had left, and I held my tongue. I took a flight back to London to our convent in Portobello. There I changed my nun's habit, which I loved, for a grey suit, black shoes and stockings. The biggest wrench to my soul was to part with my lovely white bonnet. I left with just one change of clothes and underwear, two towels and £100 in cash, but I also had a wealth of spiritual assets which have supported me throughout my life.

Out in the world I had no community to help me, no knowledge of London and, looking back, I wonder how I had the courage to do what I did. It had to be my destiny. Taking one day at a time seemed sufficient, and I was full of hope, simply trusting in Divine Providence. From the day I left the convent my motivation swept me forwards. I never wrote to any one of my superiors and I never talked about my time in the convent to my new friends. It had been a sacred time in my life and I kept silent about it. I felt myself to be still in the service of God's poor. Although I was in the world, I was still not of it. Being a nun had been too great a part of my life. I continued my spiritual exercises. Mass and daily Holy Communion were my food and drink, a necessary part of my existence. It was important to me to use my smile, which cost me nothing to give, and when given away always came back.

In London, I set about gaining admission to a school of

midwifery and was accepted by St Mary's Maternity Hospital, Commercial Road, East London. The matron was a very nice, homely woman. She asked me to become a member of staff on the 1st of January 1966. The course commenced in March but they were short of nurses, and the arrangement to help out on the maternity wards for a couple of months before my new training began suited me because I had no money. The hospital accommodation was small but to have my own little cell, after nineteen years sleeping in a common dormitory, was sheer luxury! The maternity wards were bursting with women awaiting delivery of their babies. Listening to the foetal heart was so exciting and I prayed I would never deliver an imperfect baby. I never did. I loved this new life and my studies were captivating.

After our Part 1 examination, we had to apply to another hospital to finish Part 2, and I chose St James's Hospital, Croydon, which was a small cottage hospital run by a very strict matron, who did not accept failures. I did my district midwifery on a bicycle, under the supervision of a qualified midwife. This was a blessing in disguise as the fresh air greatly improved my health. At night I would be tearing around to deliver babies, often forgetting to put my bicycle light on in my haste to get there on time. Mothers, husbands and babies had come into my life at last, and my dream was realised.

For the first time in years I was able to enjoy biting into a juicy apple and feeling freedom within my own body! Proof that if you are ill, the best remedy is to study something new. On the 31st of March 1967 I qualified and became a member of the Central Midwives Board, registration no. 182823. I was overjoyed.

On my first holiday, I went back to Autun: not to visit my friends in the convent, because that was not allowed, but to visit the old couple who had lost their suicidal son, John. While I was still a nun, he used to ask me to translate letters from an American girlfriend, whom he had met in Autun. His mother would not hear of his getting married because he suffered from epilepsy, which had started at the age of fifteen. John was an only child and simply craved love. His mother had so much fear that he didn't have the freedom to make choices of his own. One day he came to me to have a dream interpreted. Here it is:

'I dreamed I was dead and that I was being judged. A huge curtain opened. Two angels were balancing a big scales and I was perspiring because all the sins of my life were weighing in the balance against me – I could see them plainly before me when suddenly a beautiful lady appeared and in her hand she had a very small something which was placed on the other side of the scales. Lo and behold, the balance swung in my favour. I was saved!'

I talked to John and explained that he was a good Christian and in the hour of his need Our Lady would be there to rescue and comfort him. He left me, seemingly contented with my guidelines. I saw him again at Christmastime when he came to give presents to our charges and assisted at midnight Mass. He was a fervent Christian and a daily communicant. Everybody loved John because he was a good man.

I was deeply shocked when, two days after Christmas, he committed suicide. He had a huge love in his heart and suffered because this love could never be shared with the woman of his dreams. I was able to tell his heartbroken parents about his dream and help them to bear their sorrow, which was dreadful. They had no other child or caring relative. His father was in despair and his mother died later of bone cancer.

Dr Cusson, who had treated me for so long, could not believe his ears when he heard of my new studies. He was amazed that a frail person like myself could handle the job of midwife.

Back in London in 1966, I met a young Irish priest who had a late vocation, Patrick Keaveny. He was of average height, with a fair complexion and blue eyes, and I was struck by his deep faith and kindly, charismatic attitude, as well as his integrity. He was to become a Monsignor later on but I was grateful that he became my spiritual director, mentor and great friend. He told me, 'Times have changed. Women will cease to be in religious garb or living in convents. You are now needed in the world of today, to be a light of Christ, like yeast in the dough silently bearing witness to God's goodness.'

When I had finished my midwifery studies and was about to look for a job, Father Patrick asked me if I would fill in for a while as matron in a house for the aged in the East End of

London where the matron was on sick leave. I agreed, on one condition: that it was only for a couple of months, because I wanted to practise midwifery and work with mothers and children. He was as good as his word. I earned a good salary there, had a great apartment, good staff, and plenty of scope to improve standards and impart joy, but I was not in my element. Caring for the elderly had passed out of my agenda.

I applied for a job as midwife and was accepted by St Stephen's Hospital, Fulham – now the Chelsea and Westminster. I did not know London very well but a colleague directed me to a billboard in Earls Court, where I might find accommodation. I was lucky. The very first number I phoned had a bedsitter available in New King's Road, over an antique shop called Cheap and Cheerful. It is now a very posh establishment. It was a lovely family – an English lady married to an Italian, with a most delicious little daughter called Emily. My room on the top floor was very clean and, best of all, within walking distance of my work.

My year's stay in St Stephen's was a happy one. There was a homeliness about the hospital, in spite of its long, dark corridors and the nightly invasion of the big kitchen with cockroaches. The Midwifery Unit was always full and we were kept busy in the labour ward. One morning when I was in charge, an African lady was admitted in a very distressed condition. I did the usual examinations and concluded that the lady had a Bandel's ring constriction of her uterus. I phoned for the obstetrician, who came at once. My diagnosis was correct.

With no time to lose, I quickly prepared her for theatre, where the obstetrician delivered by Caesarean section a healthy male child. There was great joy, because mother and baby could both have died. The doctors and midwives had never seen the condition of Bandel's ring, where the upper and lower segments of the uterus are misbehaving. I felt very proud, for it had been one of the questions fired at me during my recent oral exams! To this day, I am enthralled by the mechanisms of labour, and indeed all muscular mechanism.

One evening I had a strange experience of another kind. It was a Friday, about seven. I had sent all the pupil midwives to supper and was sitting at the desk in the middle of a big ward of mothers and babies. All were preparing for the arrival of their husbands and families. The radio was on a small shelf on the wall behind me. Suddenly, it announced that a major plane crash had happened at Heathrow Airport. I rose from where I sat to turn up the volume so that the patients could hear, but none of them took any notice. I was surprised, but thought their minds were on other things. When the student midwives came back from supper, I told them about the air crash. At home I listened to the ten o'clock news but there was no mention of a crash. The students assured me next morning that I must have been hearing voices.

On Sunday morning a lovely lady, of about forty-two, was waiting for her baby and had asked me to deliver her. It was a breech birth so the labour was long. Her husband was waiting in the corridor outside, reading the newspaper. I asked him if there was anything strange or startling. 'Yes,' he said, 'a horrible air crash with all on board killed. One hundred and eighty people.' So the radio message had been a real communication to me. I felt quite sick – but the lady had her beautiful baby son (he was perfect) and husband and wife were jubilant. Still I could hear that radio announcement, which left me perplexed. I went home. I was to have a week off and it was lucky I did, because the incident sparked off in me a great fatigue and suffering. Why did I hear the announcement? Was there to be no escape from others' death and pain? Maybe these people needed spiritual help? Perhaps I knew somebody on that plane? I do not know but I remember praying for them.

During 1967, because my salary was so low, I decided to do some private midwifery to save a few pounds for a holiday. I worked in the Westminster Hospital in the public and private sector and loved it – but I *still* could not earn enough! In 1968 I studied trichology, which is the care of the scalp and hair, and because of my other diplomas received a better salary. In November of that year I met Joseph Toffolo.

That first meeting with Joseph Toffolo had been engineered by a couple of my work team in St Stephen's. There was always a kind of match-making conspiracy going on among the midwives. I had just returned from my mother's funeral and was working in Westminster Hospital when, to cheer me up, they set up a foursome for an evening out.

My first impression of Joseph was one of surprise. Though he looked and sounded English he was a true Italian in temperament. (He had lived in Britain since he was one year old and had completed all his schooling and studies here.) Yet here was a man of forty quite happy to be surrounded by beautiful women without any deep desire for marriage. To quote him: 'Marriage is a good institution for other people.' He was not a domestic man, nevertheless he was very domesticated. He was a romantic and remained faithful to the eternal values of beauty and proportion. He lived in rented accommodation in a Victorian house in Battersea, south London.

His treasured possessions were his books, a bust of Verdi, a gramophone, a great number of classical records, operatic scores, a radio and his dreams. He loved music, adored opera and old churches, and took a couple of months' holiday every year with his rucksack on his back – being aware of real values, he was a great traveller, loved mountain climbing and exploring ancient civilisations. Joseph's real passion was music: his genetic legacy because his father could play any stringed instrument and his sister was an accomplished violinist. Joseph wanted to study music but his cherished dreams were shattered by his mother, who objected that music had no financial benefits.

While pursuing his profession of architecture, he had written and illustrated a thesis on the design and features of the great European opera houses. He achieved a synthesis of his two great loves, opera and classical buildings. He never passed an old church without going inside. Immaculate in his appearance, he had a great sense of style. He loved to dress elegantly, whether classically as the occasion demanded or smart casual.

Always he had beautiful cravats and silk scarves of the most incredible colours. Issey Miyake shirts without collars were his great favourites. Women particularly loved the way he dressed and even children thought he looked very 'cool'. He had an incredible affinity with children, who were always asking him to sing for them.

I felt wholly inadequate as I knew nothing about opera, theatre or classical music, which was Joseph's first question to me. I was not ready to open my heart about my own dreams and ambitions. Thirty-nine years old, recently returned to the world to study and better serve humanity, I was not looking for commitment. On this note a great friendship developed.

Joseph initiated me by introducing me to music and opera. He wanted me to meet his great friend Luigi Negri, and his wife Anna, so we made up a foursome. Under a black velvet coat I wore a white blouse and a long black velvet skirt I had made myself, with the needlework skills inherited from my mother. *The Force of Destiny*, sung in Italian at Covent Garden, was my first taste of heavenly music. I then understood why Joseph looked on Verdi as his God: his tears were falling unrestrained. Joseph became my teacher in art and music. He opened my ears to sounds that I had never experienced before. Watching Joseph's tears flow during operatic performances gave me a window into his sensitive and romantic soul.

On the 27th of December 1969, thirteen months after meeting Joseph, I left London for Paris. London was extremely expensive to live in and I had always felt a magnetic pull towards the French capital, though I had not yet visited it. I telephoned Joseph in the morning to tell him of my plans. He did not seem surprised, but was disappointed that his car was in the garage and that he could not drive me. He insisted on coming with me by taxi through the snow and sleet. At the airport he produced a gift-wrapped packet. I was taken aback when I opened it and found a black enamel compact with a shamrock of marcasite inlay on the lid. I still have that compact. It is very battered, and carried with love and belongs among my treasures. At this time Joseph still did not know about my life in the convent. This would remain a secret for another two years but, at that moment, if he had begged me stay and marry him maybe I would have said yes. I am glad he did not because my tale of two cities was about to begin.

CHAPTER 6

LIFE IN PARIS

What is this life if, full of care,
We have no time to stand and stare.

No time to stand beneath the boughs
And stare as long as sheep or cows.

No time to see, when woods we pass,
Where squirrels hide their nuts in grass. . . .

A poor life this if, full of care,
We have no time to stand and stare. – W. H. Davies

It was in Paris that I found my true spiritual home. As soon as I set foot in that beautiful city a whole new energy arose (and still does) within me, a sense of well-being, a kind of reckless ness. I suppose it was here that I became liberated, broke loose from my hitherto sheltered life, tasting another aspect, or many other aspects, of love.

I gained a wealth of experience in a short time. I call it my initiation into the real world, and I count myself extremely fortunate to have found love in so many dimensions. It was like learning the complete love of God in His human form. I hardly knew anyone and it was imperative to find work to survive. At the end of the first week, I obtained an interview with the British Hospital for the post of midwife. The vacancy was not available until June or July, when the present midwife was leaving to have a baby of her own. I was accepted for the post but in the meantime still needed to earn my living.

The matron kindly furnished me with the telephone number of an agent who had English nursing training. Within a few days Mlle Berlemont had landed me a post in a Russian establishment 30 kilometres south-east of Paris in the Brie country. I was the only qualified nurse there, with responsibility for about eighty elderly Russian emigrants and staff. On my weekends off, I was replaced by a lovely nurse from Paris who had a gorgeous studio in rue d'Université. We exchanged our rooms: Liza gave me hers in Paris and she had mine in Rosay-en-Brie, together with my bicycle.

My sudden departure from London sparked more interest on the part of Joseph Toffolo, who wrote to me with an invitation to share the Oberammergau experience with him. 'Oberammergau,' he wrote, 'is a village in the Bavarian Alps in South West Germany, site of the few surviving Passion Plays. As the fulfilment of a vow made during an epidemic of plague the performance has taken place every tenth year (with a few exceptions) since 1634. It remains entirely amateur, the villagers dividing the parts among themselves and being responsible for the production, music, costumes and scenery.'

I was intrigued and my reply, by return of post, was, 'I would love to come with you, it will be my first real adventure!' However, on the eve of our departure I received a phone call telling me the midwifery post was available. When I explained about my plan for a month's holiday, they very politely told me that the vacancy could not wait. I asked for one night 'to sleep on it'. The next morning found me phoning to turn down the post in favour of the holiday. After a life of work and constraints, I thought my poor brain needed clearing of a few cobwebs! Who better to spend my first holiday with than Joseph Toffolo.

Joseph took the boat to Ostend, where we met. As the whole trip had been booked through Thomas Cook, a hired car was waiting, a tiny Renault Deux with a soft hood. Our first stop was the Hôtel de la Forge near Armentières. This hotel was very original, with a menu fit for a king. Before serving, the huge salmon was brought around the tables for approval; the other dishes likewise. It seemed a wonderful note for the start of my first real break.

After a restful night in our separate rooms and a good breakfast, we set out on our journey, stopping *en route* to drink in the sweetness of the countryside through which we passed. Joseph's excitement was contagious: he sang and together we were at ease, with a whole month to enjoy living. At Oberammergau, the Passion Play was superbly acted. The characters were carefully studied by the actors selected to play the parts of Christ, His Mother, disciples and crowds. The theatre was austere and half open to the elements, and had very uncomfortable chairs – symbols of penance, prayer and stark reality!

We spent a few days in Salzburg, where we enjoyed magnificent weather. Joseph with great pride showed me the linked squares with their typically Austrian architecture, which he had written about in his thesis. We visited the salt mines and also managed to attend a few concerts and the famous Puppet Show of *The Magic Flute*. On our return journey we took in many sights of beauty, in particular the fairy-tale castles of the mad King Ludwig II of Bavaria. His great physical beauty, his devotion to the music of Richard Wagner and his passion for building castles made him the dream king of legend. Right up my street! We visited two of them and Joseph gave Linderhof more points for its architectural purity than Neuschwanstein, although the latter castle is claimed as Ludwig's crowning achievement.

From King Ludwig's castle we took the scenic route into Italy, stopping in Venice, Verona, Milan, Torino and crossing the Galibier Pass into France. The weather was glorious, and with the car hood down we were like two students hungry for adventure. We decided to travel across the Massif-Central to visit the famous Lascaux caves, where we stood enraptured by the beauty of the paintings. The whole trip revitalised me in body, mind and spirit, and I was at last ready for the next challenge awaiting me in Paris. However, I had learned an important lesson with Joseph's help. Often I had advised mothers that their children need time to think – picking flowers, fishing for crabs or admiring glorious sunsets, painting their own images in the firmament as they watch the clouds roll by. Little ones are so receptive and thrive on these enriching experiences. Respect for life and every living creature can be instilled into their hearts. All the while I had been giving this good advice, I had been starving my own needy soul with a diet of too much hard work. Taking time to relax is important in our search for freedom: it's one of the easiest and most delightful ways to feel in touch with the intelligence of the cosmos. I had a new determination that, from now on, more laughter and recreation would be part of my agenda.

Whilst I was on holiday, all my official nursing papers had arrived from Dublin and London thanks to my spiritual friend, Monsignor Patrick Keaveny, who nudged the Irish Nursing Association into action. Mlle Berlemont had arranged an interview with the famous American Hospital in Paris which is in the 16th *arrondissement*, Neuilly, quite a select and upper-class area. I could never have landed a job at this hospital for the rich and famous without negotiating lots of red tape; but the daughters of Ireland were highly qualified and hot favourites.

Post-operative nursing was now to be my speciality, but I had to nurse some desperately ill patients, many of whom died. Fate had taken me full circle. Once more I was caring for the dying, but this time not the poorest on earth but the richest and most illustrious of God's children, whose spiritual poverty was often greater. My midwifery studies had fulfilled my dreams in part, and now I was frequently helping patients with a different kind of birth: to the next world.

*

For the first year I lived in hotels close to my work, but later on I found the most wonderful studio near the Moulin de la Galette. I called it my spaceship. It was on the top (fifth) floor, with one big french window and a balcony running along the whole width of the studio looking down on the rooftops! I was so happy. The spaceship was perfect, with an east-west orientation, ideal for me to sit on my bed and watch the setting sun, the thunderstorms, and the naked night skies studded with stars.

I worked both day and night shifts, especially loving the stillness of the night which is like a silken wrap enveloping us and taking us beyond the reach of time to the immense love of our Creator. In the night I was able to write letters and poetry and still have many daylight hours to enjoy Paris. My free spirit took flight – love and all things beautiful played a vital part in this new adventure.

In October 1970, I was given charge of a very sick lady. Mimi was forty-nine and had been ill for ten years with cancer of the pancreas. Her husband had a diplomatic post in charge of cultural affairs and the press. Every evening he would visit his wife and sit by her bed in silent grief. I admired this unique man. Later I was to learn that he had obtained every possible cure then emerging from the USA to no avail, except to prolong her suffering and his sorrow. All his wife wanted was to go home and be nursed there day and night: she did not want to die in hospital. I had been visiting Mont-Saint-Michel for the weekend, and when I returned I found

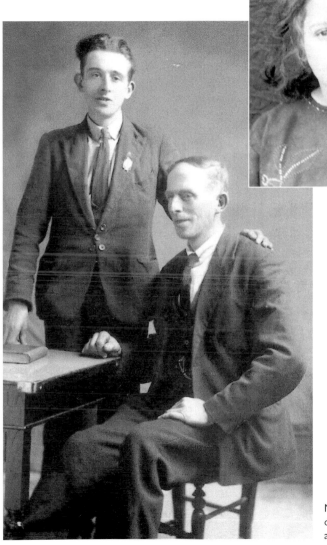

Aged five. Not long after my brother died.

My father (*seated*), for once without his hat, and my young godfather.

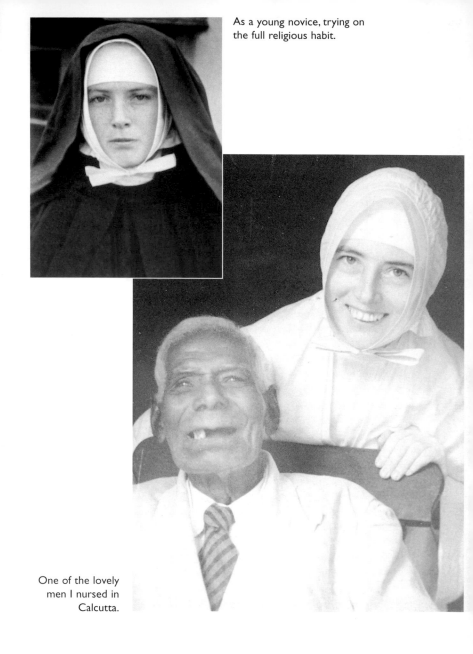

As a young novice, trying on the full religious habit.

One of the lovely men I nursed in Calcutta.

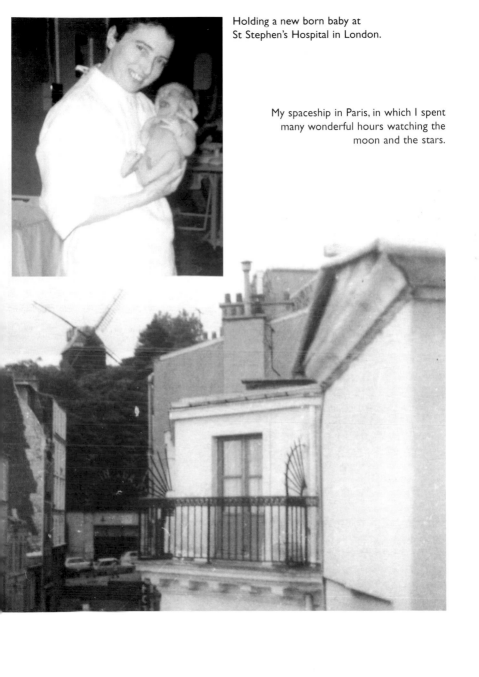

Holding a new born baby at
St Stephen's Hospital in London.

My spaceship in Paris, in which I spent
many wonderful hours watching the
moon and the stars.

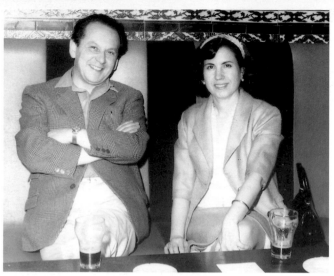

Joseph, in his thirties, enjoying a Guinness with a fellow singer.

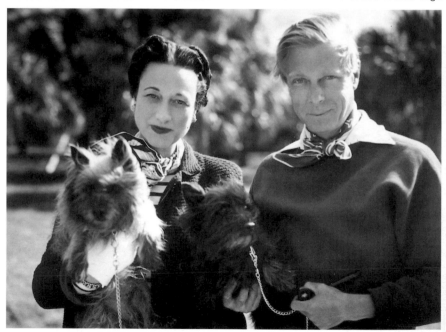

The Duke and Duchess of Windsor with two of their dogs.

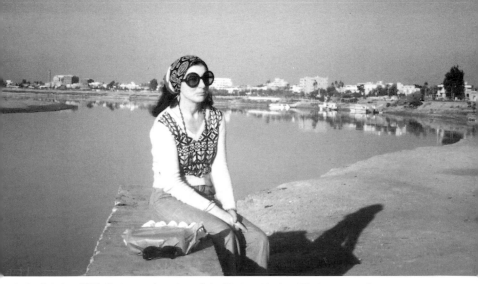

In Baghdad in 1973. Sitting at the edge of the Tigris with the 'Christmas eggs'.
In front of the famous arch of Ctesiphon in Iraq. *(Joseph Toffolo)*

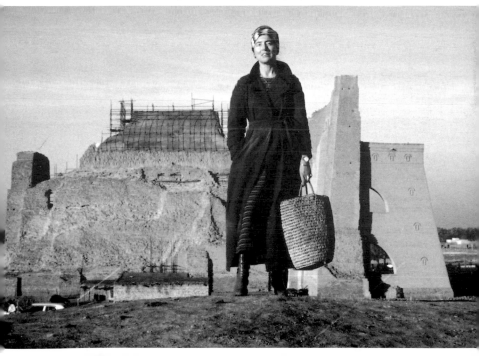

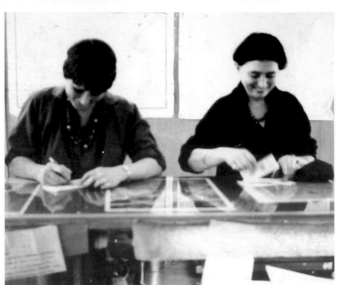

Changing money in China was an artform. Here Margaret MacDonald (*left*) and I are doing our best.

Our Chinese professor was a great teacher, and also extremely gentle.

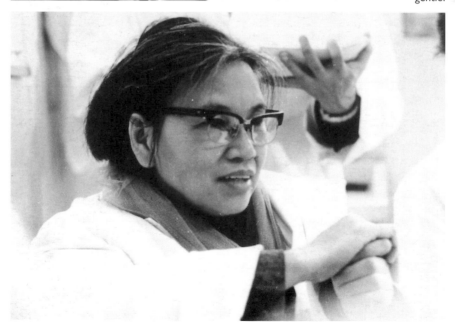

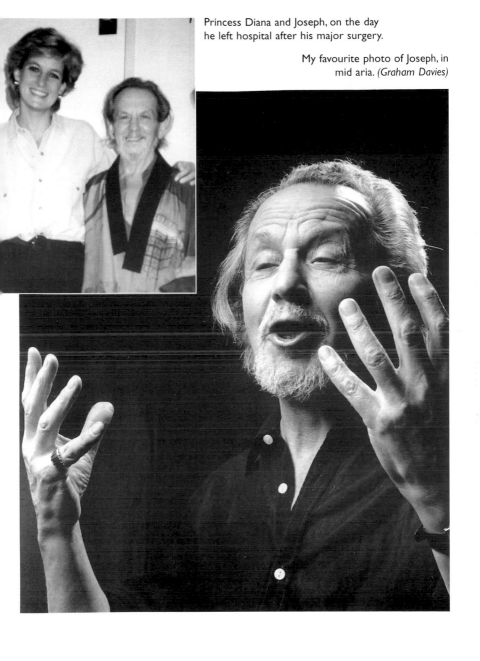

Princess Diana and Joseph, on the day he left hospital after his major surgery.

My favourite photo of Joseph, in mid aria. (Graham Davies)

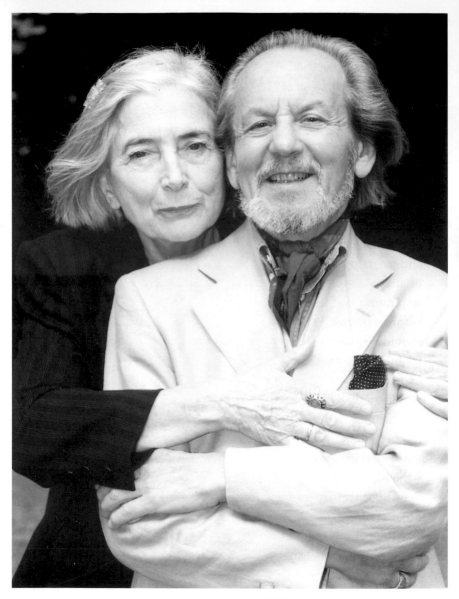

Joseph and I in Nevern Square in 1998. *(Paul Draper)*

the nursing office had received a request for me to take the night shift with Mimi for the next few weeks to help her die in peace in her own home. It was she, herself, who demanded my presence, saying that when I was on duty she did not need painkillers.

The night shift started at 11 p.m. I always arrived fifteen minutes early to have a coffee and receive the day report. On one particular Friday night Monsieur was agitated because he had seen his wife's condition worsen and was afraid that her drugs might not be adequate. He told me of his doubts and fears on my arrival. I excused myself to ascertain the cause of his worries and, having checked her temperature, pulse, respiration and blood pressure, was sure she was going to die before morning. I returned to tell Monsieur, who asked me if he should remain by her bedside. I said yes, even though he was frightened of death and his wife's death would be a shocking experience for him.

When the day nurse left, I settled Mimi and made her comfortable. Monsieur came and sat on the left-hand side of the bed, holding her hand in his. I sat opposite. All night he whispered the most loving words. I shall never forget that night – the blessedness, the tenderness, the Love. He reminisced with her about their first meeting at the fountain of St-Michel and other great moments of their life together.

About 4 a.m. he made a sign that he wanted to leave the room to smoke a cigarette. I had given his wife an injection of palfium about fifteen minutes before and she was peaceful –

then, when Monsieur released her hand and kissed it, she smiled.

Only five minutes later she sighed her last breath. Quickly I recalled Monsieur, placed a lighted candle in her hand and we both prayed in silence. While the heart-broken gentleman was busy with arrangements, I took on the sacred duty of laying out Mimi and making her look lovely using my own make-up and surrounding her bed with flowers. She looked beautiful and her husband was visibly moved.

I was invited to breakfast and after a silent coffee said goodbye to Monsieur and left. I had been with Mimi several weeks.

That morning was the 28th of October 1970, the second anniversary of my own mother's death. I had the weekend off and took the opportunity to revisit Mont-Saint-Michel. I needed a breath of pure sea air before restarting night duty at the American Hospital. When I returned Mlle Berlemont told me that a gentleman had rung several times but would not leave his name. She also asked me if I would do her a favour and sleep in her apartment to answer the telephone while she went horse-riding in the Bois de Boulogne. At about four o'clock the telephone rang. It was Monsieur: he had been desperate to find me to talk about Mimi and her recent death. He wanted me to join him for lunch at an exclusive restaurant the next day. I tried to tell him that I was on night duty but he sounded so pained that I agreed. Next morning there was no sleep for me so I wiped away the night's fatigue and dressed for lunch.

Monsieur was already there when I arrived. All the tables were reserved and the wine on our table was uncorked. Sainte Amour was the name of the wine and to this day it is my very favourite, its symbolism marking our friendship and love, which happened by accident.

One night while nursing his wife I had reached into the huge fridge for some milk to cool down my coffee when Monsieur came up behind me. Pointing out that I never ate anything, he invited me to help myself to salmon or whatever I fancied. I spun around to thank him and our lips met in a kiss. There was no warning and no lead-up to that fleeting kiss. I don't even know how it happened. I felt embarrassed but acted just like before. When I left my nursing duties at his house, I never expected to see him again. But during that special lunch this unique man told me that he felt my kiss was a holy kiss and that he loved me, which prompted me to share with him my secret about my twenty years in the convent.

Looking across the table at this handsome man and listening to his voice set my heart skipping for joy. It was like the partaking of a sacred repast by two people who had been separated for a long, long time and that lunch was a celebration of our love. Who can measure time and its mystery of how and when soulmates meet? It set the compass for the rest of our wonderful journey together. He initiated me into unheard-of delights, a foretaste of paradise. He wrote to me every day and even passed me love notes across the dinner table in restaurants. Endless surprises appeared out of nowhere when I least expected them. He introduced me to many remarkable people and showed me a new dimension to living and loving in Paris.

He adored me and I worshipped him – it was like falling in love with Christ all over again and he was in the flesh. Divine and human love had met . . . One Christmas we attended Midnight Mass in Rouen Cathedral, where I took Holy Communion. He was not a Catholic but when I got up from the communion rail he was standing behind me to kiss me and take me back to my seat. These reverential testimonies of his love I will never forget, a love that changed my life. My health was blooming and I felt healed. I rejoiced in my happiness.

It seemed nothing could destroy this precious gift. He often said, 'The only thing I ask of God is that I shall die with your hand in mine', but neither of us was ready to entertain death because we had already found Heaven!

Alas this love was to be torn from me only two years later when he died in my arms in the American Hospital. He was aged fifty-two, looking fit and handsome, and had just been admitted for cardiac investigations. My world came to an end that 2nd of August 1972.

Geneviève D'heurle, a friend of mine, was a huge support at that dreadful time. She helped prepare my beloved in his bed before he was taken to the mortuary, another day in my life which is painful to write about. That evening when I returned to my spaceship, I was desolate. I could not stop crying and in the middle of it all Joseph phoned from London. Through my tears I told him what had happened. He had rung to announce that he was going to Italy via Paris and to ask if I could find him a room. Now he was proposing that I should go with him but I told him I had already accepted the Nice flat of Rives Child (the American Ambassador) to get away from it all (he was the lover of one of my patients).

Joseph persuaded me to accompany him to Nice, as he was driving. It was the worst trip. My soul was broken and I was impossible with Joseph. Somewhere in the middle of the French countryside he stopped the car and got out, went to the boot and took out my suitcase, put it on the side of the road and very calmly told me that if I wanted to go to Nice I would have to walk because he couldn't stand me any longer. Joseph could be good for your soul! It was exactly what I needed. I begged his forgiveness and promised to behave myself. This incident gave me a new insight into the man sitting beside me. The rest of the journey was full of sympathy and we got back to being friends again. Perhaps this was the point when friendship became relationship.

In the Ambassador's flat we rested. Joseph indulged his curiosity in the vast library while I tried to come to terms with my loss amid bitter tears. When it was time for Joseph to continue his journey he would not leave me behind and suggested I come with him to Caorle, a fishing village beyond Venice where I could remain to grieve; when I was ready, he would return to fetch me.

To distract me he would show me some of the countryside,

he said. And so we travelled to Venice. Just beyond it we found the fishermen's haven which became mine. The hotel was right on the water, my room was perfect, and lying on the beach divine. When Joseph returned in a week, earlier than expected, I was washing my hair and had wrapped it in a white towel. When I opened the door to him he stood back and said, 'Oonagh, I have never seen you look so beautiful!' I told him that I had seen the man I was mourning in a dream that very morning.

Soon we were on the road, this time with more joy in our hearts and I felt that Joseph was seeing me in a different light. He took me to meet his father in his family home at Fanna in the province of Venezia. His mother had died in August 1969 and his father, who was about eighty years of age, was a very dapper gentleman. Music was his passion too and he played us some great romantic airs on his mandolin and guitar. During the First World War he dressed as an eccentric lady to avoid being conscripted into the army. He cut a youthful figure, tearing around on his bicycle, until he died at the age of ninety on St Valentine's Day.

This time of grief was very painful for me but Joseph was by my side with his truly devout friendship. We returned via Verona where we spent an evening at the opera. It was my first time in Verona and Tchaikovsky's *The Queen of Spades* was performed. We loved it and Joseph was so pleased to see me happy again.

We dallied on that holiday, neither of us wanting it to end, but work was waiting. Back in Paris, Joseph lingered for a few more days, then returned to London.

I had my own style and felt at home in my eccentric clothes. I still have a marvellous wool dress with horizontal stripes of mauve and yellow on an orange background which I wore with a big leather belt and fantastic buckle, long brown boots, with an ankle-length army mac and very large sunglasses. Often I was stopped on the Champs-Elysées and asked where I bought my clothes. If this particular outfit had a voice, it could tell many stories. I never bought cheap clothes. I would rather shop less and pay more: quality was what counted. Dorothée-Bis garments suited me and I felt good in them. Silk underwear was a must.

It was a big change from convent life and at that time the memory of the convent was fading into the past. Seven years had disappeared since I had left the convent with few possessions and little worldly experience – but I was tasting freedom and life, talking to God without having to consult the clock or answer to bells. And as for discovering the pleasure of beautiful things, I think we all know at a deep level that clothes/style are essentially nothing – it is the soul that counts!

My spaceship was shared by my friends. Of all the wonderful countries and places where I had lived, it was here in my Parisian spaceship that I enjoyed the happiest moments of my

life. At weekends I escaped, generally with a friend but sometimes alone, to explore different places: Mont-Saint-Michel;
Dijon with its great Hôtel Chapeau Rouge and its splendid
cuisine; Deauville, staying in the Hôtel Normandie, where I
loved to hire a bicycle and ride to Honfleur feeling the breeze in
my hair. What a tonic!

The man who admired my dress sense was Michel D'heurle,
a photographer who was just starting his career and was aged
about twenty-two. His wife Geneviève worked with me in the
American Hospital. We became friends and Michel commandeered me for his model. Joseph looked on him as a son and we
had many wonderful holidays together and much tasting of
music, opera and wine. Later in London, in 1987, I was to be
invited to model for another photographer, Lord Snowdon, as
one of the 'women with character' for the great fashion designer
Issey Miyake.

In France I often posed as a novelist. I wanted to avoid talking shop and being drawn into people's illnesses and gossip. I
received many invitations to the South of France and met many
well-known people in my eccentric outfits. I enjoyed the glam-
our of it all and, as you can imagine, when I received my pay
cheques I was often down to my last five francs. Of all my
religious vows, the only one I managed to keep was the vow of
hospitality – as I served Irish coffee to my friends in my spaceship!

Of the people I nursed at this time, a general from Tehran
stands out in my mind. He had been operated on for a tumour

on his lung. He could not bear to see his body scarred, so requested a dorsal incision. He seemed the most gentle of human beings – his wife was more like the general! When I used to arrive on duty at 7.30 a.m., he was waiting for me to do everything for him. He called me 'his angel in white' and invited me to visit him, if ever I went to Iran.

Another extraordinary woman, whom I nursed as she was dying, was a countess, whose son had died young. She was a writer with amazing visions of the afterlife. This lady had daily visits from her lover, an American ambassador – then about eighty years of age – who walked ten miles a day. Elegant, strong and knowledgeable, he was also an author. He was so grateful for what had been done for his countess that he offered me his superb apartment in the hills above Nice when she died. It was in this apartment that we stayed, Joseph and myself, on our way to Italy in that sad August of 1972.

I nursed another impressive lady of about eighty years of age, who was very independent. After the operation, her daughter was incredibly generous to me. Every morning (I was doing night duty at the time) she would visit her mother and then take me home to her splendid house opposite the Musée Rodin. She herself would make me breakfast of tea, toast, marmalade and fruit, then take me back to the spaceship. I felt angels were looking after me too. Years later she continued to invite me and Joseph to her country home in Provence and to music festivals. After her mother's death, I learned how wonderfully kind this lady was to a lot of other people. And her generosity knew no bounds: with her invitations came the air tickets for both of us.

One humorous patient was a Monsieur Dubonnet, who gave me a special cocktail recipe; when I asked him how he kept so youthful, he replied, '*Love* and beautiful women.' I was now working with the rich instead of the poor. Contact with wealthy and well-known people again reminded me that health and love are the greatest wealth, that rich or poor become equal in sickness and that both need medical and spiritual care.

In February 1972, Joseph Toffolo and I were having lunch with the D'heurles in the rue Duhesme in the 18th *arrondissement*, rejoicing in good French style, when the telephone rang. It was the matron of the American Hospital on the line.

'Miss Shanley, would you come immediately to take care of the Duke of Windsor? He's to be admitted at 6 p.m., for an operation in the morning.' I looked around the table for help and inspiration, for I did not want to break up the party and leave my friends. All kinds of thoughts crowded my mind and I replied, 'But, Matron, you know I am Irish and perhaps we shall not get along together.' My efforts were in vain. 'No, Miss Shanley, you must come. You are the right person – you're bilingual and the Duke needs you. We've told him about you.'

Reluctantly I gave in and said I would be there at 6 p.m. Our lunch was finished with less jubilation and I returned to my spaceship. I was somewhat apprehensive – a little nervous about my predicament. I said goodbye to Joseph, who was left to make his own way to the Gare du Nord and back to London by train. Our weekend had ended far too abruptly. By taxi, and with a somewhat heavy heart, I arrived at the hospital. I signed the register and presented myself to Matron, who indicated the Duke's room number. He was there under the pseudonym of 'Mr Smith' to protect his privacy.

CHAPTER 7

THE DUKE OF WINDSOR

*If God had meant woman to rule over man, he would
have taken her out of Adam's head. Had He destined
her to be his slave from his feet. But God took the
woman out of the man's side, for he made her to be a
helpmate and an equal to him.* – St Augustine

On entering 'Mr Smith's' room, I introduced myself to the
Prince, who was lying on the bed, fully dressed. The Duchess
was sitting by his right side, holding his hand. The Governor of
the hospital, Mr Culley, the Duke's American doctor, Dr
Antonucci, and Dr Thin the Parisian physician, sat in chairs by
the window. The Duke said, 'So you are Miss Shanley. Have
you heard of me?' 'Yes, Sir,' I said, thinking that now he was
smiling, he scarcely seemed to have changed from all those
pictures I remembered from my childhood. Then he turned to
the much-loved woman by his side; I greeted her and in turn the
doctors and Mr Culley. It was as if, in a flash, a thousand
pictures from magazines and newspapers had come to life. At
the friendly and natural charm of the Prince, my cloak of
apprehension fell away and from that minute I loved him as a
king, as a prince – and as a man who had sacrificed his throne
for the sake of love.

After the departure of the Duchess, Mr Culley and the

doctors, I proceeded with the usual pre-operative preparations. I had been put in the picture about the Prince's present illness and also the secret one, of which perhaps he guessed the gravity but never spoke of its real nature. The operation for the hernia was a success, but not the exploratory examination of the throat tumour, situated around the left carotid artery. As they feared, it was inoperable. He had been receiving treatment for some time, but now all hopes of a cure were abandoned. There only remained about six months to live and they were to be as comfortable as possible. The doctors told me, 'He has no idea of the prognosis, neither has the Duchess. At their ages it would be needlessly distressing to tell them.' I agreed with that because they had been through so much suffering already; it was better to leave them with a glimmer of hope.

The Monday night after the operation, the Duke slept well and on the Tuesday when I came on duty, he began telling me that, in so far as possible, he liked doing things for himself. I nodded my consent, not thinking too much about it, and left briefly to fetch some medication from the nursing office. I returned to find him on his feet, struggling with the drip stand and hoping to get to the bathroom in my absence. My reaction was vitriolic.

'Sir, I'll kill you for getting out of bed. You could further damage yourself and I'm responsible for you – but of course I don't mean that literally . . .'

The Duke's laughter was such that he sat down on his bed, exhausted. That moment of informality established an intimate trust and friendship between the Duke of Windsor and myself. By Wednesday, he was sufficiently recovered for the Duchess to make two visits a day. I used to look forward to the expression of pure joy and love on his face as he heard the Duchess arrive. Sidney Johnson, the faithful valet, and Giselle Duberry, the Duchess's dresser, would bring all the Duke's food in twice daily. My duties were strictly nursing and medical and keeping out of the way when the Duchess visited. On the fifth day His Royal Highness announced his intention of returning home, regardless of stitches and doctors. Out of the blue, I suddenly heard him calling me.

'Oonagh, I am going home today because I cannot bear to be separated from Wallis another night. It's the first time in our married life that we have been separated for so long. Would you care to come home with me for a few days until this wretched wound is healed?' I replied, 'Sir, this is a deviation from normal practice but since you're on the Board of Governors, you have only to voice your request and I'll come home with you.'

Everything went according to plan, and the next afternoon I followed him and the Duchess into a big limousine with tinted windows, driven by his personal chauffeur, Mr Wilson. We sped along the Bois de Boulogne and through the grilled gates of no. 4, rue Champs d'Entrainement. It was here that the Windsors had lived in their exile since 1953, when the city of Paris and the French Government paid them the delicate compliment of offering them this grace and favour residence at a nominal rent, together with special residential status exempting them from income tax. In the huge entrance hall, twenty-five members of staff, all smiling, were gathered to welcome their prince and master back home.

A glass and gilt lift took the Duke, Duchess and myself to the first floor. On entering his bedroom, one was immediately assailed by a great splash of scarlet, blue and gold in the otherwise quiet room. The tapestry of his royal coat of arms hung directly above the large double bed with the motto: 'Honi soit qui mal y pense.' On the second floor was the magnificent scarlet, black and gold Napoleon III Suite which the Duchess had prepared for me. Later, when I settled the Duke for the night, my thoughts were on the incredible fact that I, a forty-two-year-old Irish nurse trained in Dublin, London and France, and with a long history of nursing the poor in India and France, should now be sleeping in an ornate bed with a gilt upright telephone beside it, so that the ex-King Edward VIII could summon me to his side. The most famous and romantic figure in recent royal history was totally entrusted to my medical care.

He began the next day with the question he was to ask every morning till his death: 'Is the Duchess awake yet?' If she was, he would say to his black and white pug who slept on his bed, 'Come on, Diamond, move, we must go and see the Duchess.' Then, having insisted on attending to himself without my help, he would emerge from his bathroom, shaved, brushed and smelling of talc – he always used water to smooth his hair. He wore the most stylish striped cotton nightshirts, hand-made by the household's seamstress, mid-calf-length with long sleeves and mandarin collars. Then, in his dressing gown, he would go straight to his wife's bedroom. Diamond would follow, eager to greet the Duchess's matching pug, Gen Seng.

'They miss each other too,' the Duke explained. 'Gen Seng always slept on the Duchess's side of our bed and Diamond on my side, but since I've had this damn throat trouble it seemed pointless to spoil everyone's sleep. So Gen Seng goes off with Wallis to get some good nights, and old Diamond sticks it out with me.'

Everything else that happened on that first Saturday marked for me the regular pattern of the Windsors' daily lives – a reassuring pattern the Duke strove to keep to until the end. After their first hour together, they would meet again in the intimate drawing room separating their bedroom suites for the American-style combination of light breakfast and lunch – brunch – served to them on table trays. It never varied: lightly scrambled eggs topped with wafer-thin slices of bacon, toast and tea. Later the Duke would return to the desk in his bedroom, dealing with an always large correspondence to pass on to his secretary, John Utter. He would make his daily telephone calls, dealing with his private affairs, locally and internationally. The Duchess's dresser, Giselle, was devoted and loyal; as was Sidney, the valet on whom the Duke fondly relied. Sidney had been with him for thirty-two years, taken on as a fifteen-year-old trainee, when the Duke was Governor of the Bahamas.

On the day after my arrival, I went to the first-floor drawing room where the Duke and Duchess were having brunch. He wore a red carnation in his buttonhole and the Duchess told me, 'They're his favourite flower and now we have the smallest carnation in the world – for you – for bringing him safely back to us.' She handed me a small box. On the velvet lay a miniature carnation with carved ivory petals surrounding a sapphire centre, its leaves and stem fashioned in smaller sapphires and diamonds to make a brooch. 'The Duke designed it for me,' said the Duchess, 'and now we want you to have it as a token of our gratitude for coming home with us to care for him.' The Duke added, 'And we want you to promise that if ever we need you again, you'll come back.' I promised I would and said that I could not find enough words to express my thanks. 'You, Oonagh, short of words?' the Duke teased. 'Well, find your words quickly as I intend staying up for dinner tonight and we'd like you to join us.'

At 6 p.m. I went upstairs to get ready. As I was starting to get a home of my own together, I was fascinated by the style and taste of that superb house. Even my guest bathroom was unlike any other. I knew I'd never be able to afford to emulate it but I noticed, for instance, that there was no sanitary holder but instead separately folded leaves of paper in a silver dish! I changed into a tailor-made red, black and white tartan skirt with side buttons from waist to ankle and pinned the jewelled carnation on my yellow blouse. At 7 p.m. I joined the Duke and Duchess for aperitifs. The Duke always asked me to taste his Scotch in case it was too strong. The Duchess had a small dry martini; they both drank very little. Then, sending for Sidney, the Duke asked us to excuse him for a few moments.

Soon he reappeared, looking absolutely stunning in a formal suit of Black Watch tartan. 'Look, Oonagh,' he said. 'I love the tartan so much that when I saw your splendid skirt, I thought I'd keep you company and, but for this damn throat, I'd have played the pipes too!' Indicating a swirl, he led his wife and me down to dinner in the formal dining room with its blazing fire.

Above the mantel hung an arresting portrait of the Duchess, done in oils. The table linen was so fine you could have used it for bridal handkerchiefs. Sometimes the polished table was covered with a cloth, sometimes set with place mats. On every occasion I ate with them, there was a different, priceless dinner service. The Duchess liked individual plates – which told much of her individuality! Of all the delicious meals I remember most the quail – the Duke's favourite – and a carrot purée (I disliked carrots until I tasted them prepared like that). The Windsors often invited me to dine with them and it was a marvellous experience because they were so easy to be with. They had a harmony together and included everyone in it. I often wondered why so many unkind things had been said about them.

One afternoon the Duchess showed me the formal ground-floor drawing room, hung with paintings of the Duke's family: his great-grandmother Queen Victoria, grandparents Edward VII and Queen Alexandra, and parents George V and Queen Mary. The imposing room was filled with a fragrance of white lilies and orchids. I turned to the Duchess and said, 'Everywhere you look – it's so beautiful here, your Royal Highness.' (Everyone in the house gave her the royal title.) The Duchess smiled, answering quietly, 'I made up my mind that David should always live as a king – wherever we were.' It seemed that the Duke had also made up his mind that his wife should always be treated as the Queen he had been unable to make her. Though his family refused to confer royal status on her – and he once told me that was his 'still open wound' – he treated her as though she were more royal than himself. He wouldn't even let her handle any used money. Every day he gave her a wad of newly minted French banknotes.

On the last day of his recuperation, I thanked him for all his kindness and unthinkingly lapsed into French. He stopped me: 'Oonagh, no! Don't speak in French. It's a beautiful language, especially for a woman, but with me please always speak in English.' Suddenly I remembered the land he had left, the English voices he so rarely heard, and again it brought forcefully home to me how, in so many ways, his exile grated against his very sense of identity. England was not that country just across the Channel; for him it had become a truly faraway place. At the same time, it was the cultural foundation of all that he held to be important, all that defined him – yet it was no longer his land. I vowed right then to speak only his native tongue, thinking how difficult it must be for him to be denied his birthright, his beloved English language.

Only five weeks later he did need me, when he entered the last phase of his illness. I was saddened when I saw him again – thinner, weaker, his voice hoarser. When the Duchess took me back to the same guest suite, she said, 'I've arranged for hot drinks and sandwiches to be left in your room every night . . . in case . . .' Her slightly American, low voice trailed off unhappily.

At dinner that night she said sadly, 'I have this lasting sense of loss that we could never have a child. Above everything we both wanted one but, you see, I had to have a hysterectomy only twelve months after we married.'

As it was, without a child, you could see they'd developed an almost parental caring for each other. Most accounts I had read of their love story suggested it was he who did all the loving, while she just accepted it. That wasn't true. She ran that household lovingly, planning each detail for his every need and comfort. But in their last weeks together, it did seem to me that probably all his married life he'd tried to protect her so much that he'd barely given her a chance to express many of her true reactions. As he became increasingly ill, with coughing spasms and slight fevers, the first thing he wanted to know was if he would be able to get up for dinner with the Duchess – even though he could scarcely eat.

Whenever he couldn't join her, he wanted her secretary to ensure that some of her American friends would either be invited to dine or alerted to ask her out.

'Wallis loves people, parties and good conversation,' he told me. 'The very last thing I want is that she should be at all worried about me.' (The Duke was so conscious of the odour from the tumour that he hated to incommode anyone with it.) 'She makes everyone laugh and I want that to go on.' To keep the Duchess company, he relied especially on Lady Grace, Countess of Dudley, the widow of one of his closest friends from his Oxford days.

As the Duke began to suffer slight haemorrhages from his throat, he still insisted the Duchess should not be told. He liked to know that Mr Clement, her make-up artist from Elizabeth Arden, had been to visit her and that Alexandre, her hairdresser, was still coming three times a week. Nothing should be cancelled because of him.

By this time, a month before his death, daily bulletins on his health were being sent to Buckingham Palace. The Queen and Prince Philip, due to make a state visit to France, and to be joined by Prince Charles, were planning a private call on the Windsors on Thursday, the 18th of May – but on the 10th he had his first cardiac arrest. That night I had the evening off and dined with friends in the Latin Quarter. When I returned at midnight, I found the Duke agitated; a minute later, he had a total cardiac collapse. I was alone and had no time to waste. I ran to my room, grabbed an ampoule of cortisone from my medical bag, quickly injected it intravenously and commenced cardiac massage. The cocktail of prayers, medicine and action worked. His pulse returned and his blood pressure registered again.

When I was satisfied, I phoned his doctor, Dr Thin, informing him of the crisis and asking him to bring his ECG machine. Dr Thin dashed across Paris and after a thorough examination of the Duke, left around 3 a.m., promising an early morning visit, with Dr Jacquin, to install an intravenous drip of the vitamins and minerals necessary to maintain normal cardiac function.

When the Duke awoke the next morning, he remembered what had happened and his first question was: 'You haven't told Wallis?' 'No, Sir,' I replied. Then he said, 'So, Miss Shanley, you saved my life last night – it appears I was dying.' This being the early seventies, I joked that my response was speeded by the hashish I had smoked that night. He found this very amusing. (From then on, whenever I was going out for the night, he would call out, 'Don't overdo the hashish tonight!') He asked, 'How many days before my family comes?' 'Eight, Sir, but you'll be feeling better by then.' 'I'm determined to,' he said. 'I'm very fond of Charles. He asked to spend an evening with me here, when he was on a state visit to Paris – the only time two Princes of Wales have met in hundreds of years, you know. Had a long talk. He's a fine fellow – splendid young man.'

These are my diary entries for the days leading up to the Queen's visit:

May 13th Saturday – Better form – Coramine continued.

May 14th Sunday – Good form. T.P.R. [temperature, pulse, respiration] normal – ate a good dinner.

May 15th Monday – Continued to feel better.

May 16th Tuesday – Treatment to maintain good heart function.

May 17th Wednesday – Condition stabilised.

May 18th Thursday – Treatment stopped, drip taken down at the Duke's request, did not want to receive Her Majesty hung on a drip. Duke not too good, feeling tired and nervous but still very strong mentally.

The Queen came. I was the only other person present.

On the morning of the 18th of May, tired and stressed as he was, the Duke of Windsor knew exactly what he wanted to wear, as he always did. The whole household was atremble with excitement.

Laurence, the make-up artist, had come to the Duchess to prepare her, and Giselle Duberry came to me with this request: 'Oonagh, could you ask HRH to give Laurence his blessing?' I approached HRH (the Duke) with the request and to my joy, he replied, 'Oonagh, I will do this for you – after all he has been a decent chap, coming whenever the Duchess needs him.' In return Laurence lavished his expertise on me by giving me a facial for the Queen's visit. I was touched by the sick man's effortful gesture, amid the hurry and flurry of the preparations to receive the Queen. When Miss Schultz, his secretary, phoned me later I was still with the Duke.

'What is that about?' he asked.

'Sir,' I answered. 'Miss Schultz is telling me to wait in a side room until the visit is over—'

'You will do no such thing. I want you right beside me.'

So that was that. I knew he was worried that though he was better, he might have another sudden haemorrhage. At 4.15 p.m. in the informal drawing room, I waited with him. He was seated in his wheelchair, dressed in dark trousers and a blue polo-neck sweater to match the cornflower blue of his eyes. In spite of his illness there was an aura of light about him – his charisma was palpable. He knew the Duchess would bring only the Queen upstairs first, and as Her Majesty came in the Duke stood up – a great effort for him – and said, 'My dear Lilibet,' and kissed her on both cheeks. The Queen asked him how he was feeling. 'Not so bad,' he said gamely, managing a brilliant smile for the niece whose life he had changed so drastically by his abdication.

He presented me to the Queen, explaining, 'This is Oonagh, who takes such care of me that I like to keep her by my side. She's Irish, but is not here to shoot me but surrounds me with loving care.' It was so typical of his marvellous consideration and kindness, but that one effort tired him and he remained seated when Prince Philip arrived and shook hands very warmly. As the Duchess brought Prince Charles in, his face lit up and he started asking him about the Navy, flying and riding. There was much affection between the two of them, but after a few minutes I saw the Duke's throat convulse and he began coughing. He motioned me to wheel him away. The

Royal Family stood up and left. I had the feeling that this was his way of avoiding any formal goodbyes. It had all been brief, immensely cordial and very important to him, but he had no reserve of strength left.

That night he had more distress, when his dog Diamond suddenly refused to stay in his room and whimpered and scratched to be let out. He had only another ten days of life left to him and, though growing weaker, he was more or less contented except that he frequently asked about Diamond, but wouldn't hear of anyone bringing the dog to him, saying, 'He'll come back when he wants to.' Friday, the 26th of May, was the first morning he didn't try to get up at all, allowing Sidney and myself to do everything for him. That evening his temperature soared and he was on an intravenous drip, though he seemed scarcely aware of it. In spite of a sedative, he lay with his eyes open, semi-delirious and muttering – and then his eyes brimmed with tears. I kept cooling his forehead and moistening his lips but his agony was not in his body, it was in his soul. Human warmth and touch often comforts dying patients, so I lay on the coverlet beside him and put my arm around him, and he grew quieter. Tears filled his eyes again and he said something about 'England . . . not far away . . .' and then, 'the waste . . . the waste not giving a chap a decent job to do'.

In all the conversations he had with me in the previous deteriorating days, he'd said, several times, how much he'd longed to be given a 'worthwhile job' for his own country, and a title for his beloved. Now, as he lay there, so clearly in great grief, I thought of his royal and religious upbringing – like an indoctrination – and the torment the decision to abdicate must have brought him. I couldn't know if he was reliving it – where his thoughts had gone – but his distress made me cradle his head on my shoulder – anything to bring some peace to his face. I kept murmuring his Christian name, 'It's all right, David, I'm here, David, we're all here,' hoping my voice might mean whoever he wanted it to be. At 3 a.m. he drifted into sleep. I switched off the shaded lamp, leaving only the bathroom light to filter through the slightly open door, and settled myself in an armchair to read. I was used to such long stretches of the night, but was totally unprepared for the sickening thud and crash that shattered the silence.

It came from the bathroom and as I leapt up and went in there, it happened again, this time followed by a rasping croak. I realised that some night creature was hitting against the window, probably attracted by the light. The noise set my heart thumping and I went to make sure it hadn't disturbed the Duke. Then several birds began croaking and I wished they would stop. It was now 3.45 a.m. I had been monitoring the Duke – not at all sure he would live much longer – so I woke Giselle, in case I needed assistance while I telephoned the doctor. 'What on earth are those birds making that horrible noise?' I asked her and she said, 'Oh, it's the *corbeaux*' (which I translated as ravens). I'd never heard them in the night before. Then I remembered the shiny black ravens I'd often seen in the garden and all the ominous legends, learned in childhood, came to my thoughts – the fatal ravens consecrated to the Danish war god – the ravens in *Macbeth*, croaking their warning of royal death. I knew England and the royal ravens had come for him.

It doesn't do for a night nurse to allow herself to become imaginative nor, even today, do I think I was. I simply looked at the royal coat of arms pinned to the wall above the bed, and the face of the man who had once been a king, and thought, *We are all equal in suffering*. Without sleep, I stayed with the Duke for nearly seventy-two hours, grateful to see his mental anguish subside, the fever diminish, the smile on his face when the Duchess came in. He was so brave in his suffering.

By now the Duchess was fully aware of how ill he was, in spite of the fact that even up to six hours before he died, he tried to tell her he didn't feel 'too bad'. On that Friday, after she'd kissed him good-night, there was a persistent scratching at the door and – Diamond came back! 'Diamond!' I heard the Duke say weakly. 'Oh, you're the most faithful of friends.' He slept that night, his hand on the dog's head. Throughout Saturday, the last day of his life, both the Duchess and Diamond were with him. The Duchess wanted to stay up all night. 'No, darling,' he told her, 'I shall soon be asleep. Get some rest, please.'

Until 10 p.m. Sidney kept vigil with me and we said the Act of Contrition and Our Father together. The Duke opened his bright blue eyes and looked at me. 'Oonagh, am I going to die?' I reassured him that we were praying for him, that he would not suffer – he knew he was going to die – and a few hours later, at 2.20 a.m., he slipped away quietly under the cover of night, just as he had left England, his native land.

Darkness was his companion then, but through this trial he was helped by myself and a colleague from the American Hospital, Julie Chattard, from Baltimore. She was one of the two nursing friends who covered for me when I was off duty, and I had enlisted her help on the night the Duke died. Together we kept the torch of love burning brightly for him who gave up his kingdom for love. We witnessed the sight of relief and look of peace that descended upon him: he was home at last. I thought that if I never had another patient, the privilege of knowing and caring for this unique man would have made all my life's work worth while.

I smoothed his brow and cleaned his face. After a few minutes, I fetched the Duchess. At his bedside she said, 'My David', and kissed his forehead. Then cupping her hands gently round his face, she said again, 'My David – you look so lovely.' Her quietness was much sadder than tears. As Giselle took her back to her room, she looked an old lady – though a proud one – but so alone. Giselle and I both cried for her. We couldn't help it.

A week later, at the Duchess's invitation, I went to England to attend the Duke's funeral at St George's Chapel, Windsor. In London, a letter from Giselle awaited me on Buckingham Palace notepaper. 'As you know, the Queen has invited the Duchess to stay here,' she wrote. 'And everyone is being so very kind to us.' I keep that letter with all my mementoes of the Duke, whose love story made history.

The years that followed the Duke's death were unspeakably lonely for the Duchess. This period could fill many pages and could be compared to Dante's vision of Hell. She was a martyr at the hands of greedy people.

The Duke died as he lived, not wanting to be a burden to anyone, but his love for Wallis had not diminished one iota. His greatest concern, those last weeks of his life, was that the Duchess should continue her life as usual and be spared his suffering. That was the sole reason for the supreme effort he made in appearing strong when the cancer in his throat would not allow any respite. I admired his fortitude – he was the great romantic hero, perhaps the last, in our time. His love and his confidence in Wallis proved that his abdication was justified. And it is a great pity that such a noble soul was not granted at least some of his wishes. In his death he is restored to his rightful place in history, that of King Edward VIII, and takes his place in the gallery of British sovereigns.

CHAPTER 8

MARRIAGE

Marriage is the curse of propinquity.

– Joseph Toffolo

In the summer of 1973 Joseph, with his itchy feet and yearning to explore faraway places, accepted the challenge of a job as a consultant architect in Baghdad for a period of six months. One night in Paris, I received a phone call asking me if I would like to share the experience with him.

Later in the year I returned to London for a visit and Joseph, on his two knees, asked me to marry him. Both of us had mixed feelings about marriage. When I asked Joseph, 'What is love?' he replied, 'Love is a bond.' To me, love does not erect barriers or create divisions. Tenderness and gentleness walk hand in hand. Where there is love there is no fear. I used to tease him about his intentions in asking me to marry him before accepting the contract to Baghdad, since travelling in that Muslim country as two single people would have been difficult, if not impossible. Joseph recently wrote in answer to the questioning of a mutual friend:

> After a prolonged friendship-courtship, lasting about four years, I decided it was time to get married to Oonagh (if she would have me). Throughout this period she had always been a faithful, devoted and generous companion. Personally I do not think the decision

was entirely expedited by my proposed six-month contract in Baghdad. After all, more than half the time I had known her she had been working in Paris, whilst I had remained in London. I do admit that it had some influence on the decision but to what extent, I cannot say, though I must add that without Oonagh I would not have stayed in Baghdad!

On the 8th of December 1973, Joseph and I were married in Forest Hill, South London by my friend, Monsignor Patrick Keaveny, whose advice was important to me and nearly always followed. He had encouraged me in my friendship with Joseph. For the wedding ceremony I wore a long ivory-white dress bought in Paris and a generous length of matching white silk which I fashioned into a turban fastened by my royal brooch. Over the dress I wore my own creation, a pale blue cape which I had finished at 3 a.m. on that morning. We chose our friend Julie Chattard as bridesmaid and invited thirty of our 'inner circle' to join us.

Marriage, for me, is a permanent form of monogamous, erotic relationship rather than an institution, and holds a deep spiritual meaning. Lovers who celebrate their marriage ceremony are participating in a sacred covenant – and I do not mean ecclesiastical sacredness. I chose the 8th of December as it was on this date twenty-five years before that I made my first religious vows and it seemed appropriate to link these two solemn dates in my life.

The important thing, to me, is to allow love into one's life, to turn towards it. Then, if one love dies (that of my 'Monsieur' in Paris), another will take its place (Joseph Toffolo) – whether human or Divine in form. We only have to realise love is all around us and within us, as Annabella, a French actress, once said: 'J'ai passé toute ma vie être amoureuse, amoureuse de la nature, amoureuse des animaux, amoureuse de la vie, et je fête chaque Printemps comme un miracle.' (I have passed my whole life being in love, in love with nature, in love with animals, in love with life, and I celebrate each springtime as a miracle.)

When we build a relationship (whether with God or with a human partner), the *act* of turning the heart towards the beloved, with recognition, waters the root of love. Then one can receive its fruits: peace; joy; silence; contentment.

Marrying someone is perhaps the highest, loveliest and hardest task that a man or woman can undertake: to control the current of erotic emotions and direct them only towards each other; not once but 'unto seventy times seven', to give each other that supreme joy, that foretaste of Paradise. The difficulty is guarding against the curse of routine and taking each other for granted. My recipe for a happy marriage is to repeat often 'I love you' to your partner, and to feel the silken thread uniting you both with the universe. 'My Beloved to me and I to Him who feedeth among the lilies' (Solomon), was the expression of my love for Joseph.

Of course, sometimes sparks fly and tempers boil over but I would try never to let the sun go down on my anger. I would go for a walk or soothe my ragged nerves by taking a relaxing bath and then shortly afterwards be able to say about the

difference of opinion, if I were to blame, I am sorry. You know
I love you . . .

On the 12th of December 1973, Joseph and I left for Baghdad.
Our belated honeymoon took place over many countries in
June and July of 1974. Joseph's six-month contract was to act
as liaison architect between a Scottish firm of engineers in
co-operation with an English firm of architects, and a Baghdad
architect. The project was extensions to three villages within a
30-mile radius of Baghdad. Housing needed to be designed, as
well as community buildings, restaurants and dormitories for
students. Arriving at Baghdad airport, we were met by the
engineers' representative, who warmly welcomed us and
whisked us off to our hotel. We made friends with a very
charismatic manageress named Agnes, who spoiled us. On
the 19th of December we left our friendly hotel and took up
married quarters on the banks of the Tigris in an apartment
block facing the President's Palace across the river. Our accommodation was on the first floor and consisted of an enormous
living-dining area, with two double bedrooms, a kitchen, bathroom and separate WC. There was a huge terrace which we
seldom used, because we could not appear in shorts or semi-
clothed. It was not allowed because of the sensitive position
opposite the President's Palace. We were under constant
surveillance – at least that's what we were told. This did not
bother us in the least: we knew nothing about the political

hotbed we had landed in, certainly not yet – that was a lesson for later on.

On Christmas Day 1973, we had absolutely no food in the house and decided we would eat out after a long walk. About fifteen minutes into our promenade, we heard voices and commotion. I persuaded Joseph to follow the sound and investigate. We arrived at a barrier where the sale of eggs was taking place through a grille. On our approach silence descended on the clamouring crowd. We were asked if we would like some? A young man handed us a tray of twenty-four of the most beautiful eggs. We paid a nominal price and returned to our apartment. On the way back we stopped for Joseph to immortalise the eggs on camera. I still have the photograph of myself and the famous Christmas eggs on the banks of the River Tigris. Here was the first example of Iraqi hospitality, which was to be repeated constantly during our stay and created loved and cherished memories.

To Arabs, travelling is synonymous with hospitality, and hospitality in their tradition has always been something more than a duty. It is a form of godliness for which a man must strive (as it was for my own father). An Arab family feels incomplete until a guest arrives to be entertained. In Iraq, in 1973, tourism had a meaning beyond economics or culture: it was an opportunity for self-fulfilment and private happiness. Our great joy and privilege was to share in the life of this rare breed of people, so handsome, so noble and so generous. We had access as spectators to their most sacred mosques and to their age-old wisdom. Every day at noon, and again at sundown, the call to prayer rang out. People stopped in their tracks to acknowledge Allah. Many prostrated themselves before Him. I was struck by the importance both Muslims and Christians attach to prayer. Though, while Muslims follow a set form of prayer, Christians follow ritual and liturgy. There was no vandalism, no stealing. I wore my special piece of royal jewellery without a second thought for its value or its safety. And I took care to wear mostly long skirts and keep my head covered. With my husband to care for, my life now seemed charmed with ease and grace, well away from hectic routine. The climate in Iraq is semitropical, the central and south-eastern areas characterised by a cold to moderate winter and a long dry summer, though in northern Iraq I believe it is cold, with snow and long winters and moderately hot summers. The language of the people was Arabic, though at that time English was taught as a second language in all the schools.

These were exciting times, discovering the magic of a thousand and one nights together. Joseph worked from 8.30 a.m. to 12.30 when he came home for lunch, and then again from 4.30 to 8 p.m. My days were happily spent shopping, cooking and waiting for his return. Visiting the souks was a favourite pastime and I so enjoyed communicating with the local people and playing with the children. There was a taxi service; several people shared the same taxi – which went at breakneck speed – life was never dull! In the fruit market I met a young boy who was the son of one of the stall owners. He insisted on carrying my shopping and when special delicacies came from France, he would phone and tell me that my country's best food had arrived. I was never short of anything – even brandy and whiskey was put under the counter for me. For some reason they thought I was French, and only the best was good enough for the French.

Because we were not British, we were refused membership of the All British Club, but Hisham Munir, Joseph's boss, gave us a glowing reference and personally sent a letter advising the Alwiya Club to enrol us as members. It was the upper-crust Iraqi club with every possible luxury and an amazing swimming pool. This was our greatest blessing and every afternoon we spent an hour or more here, content that the Iraqi people had taken us to their hearts.

Our trip out to Ctesiphon in Salman Pack, with its famous unsupported brick arch (the greatest in the world), was captured on camera by Joseph. Babylon was a little disappointing, as the hanging gardens had disappeared with the ravages of time. Only vestiges of its past grandeur, like the Great Lion of Babylon, remained. Basra, with its surrounding marshes, was the most evocative for us. Nearby Al-Qurna, where the Tigris meets the Euphrates, is the legendary spot of the Garden of Eden, with its famous old tree, called Adam's tree. We touched its ancient trunk and sat on the terrace of the one and only small hotel/restaurant, musing on the sacredness of the spot and drinking in its past. We thought, too, of our own destiny as man and wife. There was a mystery and stillness about the place. It felt so right that this should be the Garden of Eden and that we should be sharing it hand in hand.

Joseph told me that nowadays Basra is considered one of the most important cities of Iraq and it links the country with the outside world by sea. At that time, on the surrounding marshes, people lived on boats made from reeds and roofed in the most exquisite designs like miniature palaces. In the evening the marshes lit up with their fairy lights and the whole scene was one of indescribable beauty.

We had taken a sleeper on the night train from Baghdad, which was very comfortable – a far cry from my journeys across India!

Arriving at Ur railway station in the morning, we were harassed by a 'tourist agent' and reprimanded for taking photographs of soldiers walking on top of a railway carriage. The 'tourist agent' was surprisingly curious about us and insisted on seeing our papers. Joseph found this highly irregular. He said the man was obviously a policeman in disguise, although it was never admitted. When we took a cab to the historical site of Ur, some miles away, to save time, he insisted on coming with us. Be our guest by all means – nice to return the compliment for all the hospitality we had received! Besides, we were beginning to understand it was easy to find yourself 'inside' if too much independence in these matters was shown.

We were enraptured by Ur, the centre of Sumerian civilisation, where we saw the great sixty-foot ziggurat, a temple tower built in 2,000 BC, a place of peace and extraordinary hidden energy. At the ziggurat pyramid, which had been extensively restored, we wanted to climb the magnificent single-flight staircase but it was not permitted. Joseph was sorely disappointed: he loved climbing and walking on the very edge of time.

It was clear that our 'tourist agent' did not trust us, and cameras were dangerous toys. We were accompanied back to Ur railway station, during which time Joseph made one of his outspoken remarks about the large standing army in Iraq. (These remarks of his alarmed me, for I knew many Iraqis had disappeared for less, and at home I was always relieved when he returned safe and sound.) However, on this occasion, his remark was dismissed with a 'humph'. At the railway station we parted with the 'tourist agent' on the most amicable terms.

Back in the city of a thousand and one nights, we enjoyed its special magic – private candlelit dinners with the most delicious and varied meats and sweetmeats. A whole lamb, spiced and herbed, cooked on the spit, was a festive favourite. One particular banquet took place in a sunken garden of unreal beauty and the spectacle of belly-dancers and the music was a delight for the senses. The cool of this garden on a hot evening made me dream of the Garden of Eden.

The great heat of July and August was approaching. In June the temperatures were already soaring to 100 degrees Fahrenheit. Joseph's contract was terminating and it was time to think of moving on. After some debate, we decided to make an overland trip back to London instead of a direct flight. This belated honeymoon lasted about eight weeks in all. The journey took careful planning and was preceded by a two-week tour of Iran. We took a bus from Baghdad, going east to cross the frontier at Khanagin and cherished a tender memory: whilst waiting at the bus station a blind man sang us a song. What better farewell could one expect?

CHAPTER 9

TRAVELS IN THE MIDDLE EAST

Marriage is at once a concession and a demand, a giving and a receiving. There must be constant thought for the other partner. Marriage is also the strongest educative factor in the whole school of Life and like all school, Life is no idle game. – Von Scheffer

At the frontier we were stopped by the Iraqi army, who insisted on searching our bags and checking cameras. They seemed to be very serious about the whole thing and at the time, we did not understand why. But from Baghdad to Tehran, one could feel the political unrest which prevailed at the various places we stopped. We became chatty with a group of dubious-looking Pakistanis, who described themselves as 'merchants'. The most charismatic of them spoke English fluently. An amicable exchange developed *en route* to Tehran, and upon reaching this exciting city, we all dismounted from the bus.

The English-speaking Pakistani gentleman volunteered to take us to a hotel in town and promptly helped to load our baggage on to a kind of sledge which was dragged along by hand at a furious speed. The penny dropped that we were about to bid farewell to our luggage for good, so we ran after it as fast as we could, and managed to keep pace. We arrived at the 'hotel' – a haunt obviously full of thieves and a real den of iniquity, not to mention poor hygienic standards. There was a presence of evil in the unsavoury characters wandering around in its dark, candlelit corridors. We said goodbye to our 'guide' and fled (with our luggage) to find a more salubrious shelter for the night. Eventually we found a modest pension where, curiously, four British truck drivers were staying. One of them recounted many adventures of his transcontinental trips and spoke of the unique lunar landscape in Iran, east of Tehran.

We wanted to contact General Adjudani – the gentle Iranian who had been my patient at the American Hospital in Paris. The manager of the pension was quick in finding his phone number and a moment later the General's wife was speaking to us herself. The General, who was a handsome man with a brilliant smile, invited us to a splendid lunch with him and his daughter in the French Club. Much caviare and champagne flowed. The next night he invited us to a grand party of international VIPs in his own palatial mansion. Again the finest champagne and wines were served, with an extravagant spread of fruits, meats, fish and jellies to satisfy every taste.

The morning after this great party we were sleeping in, when a loud knocking on our door brought us swiftly back to consciousness. It was the police – some valuable rugs had been stolen the night before from the pension.

'Where were you last night?' they demanded. We told them that we were at General Adjudani's party – and with hats in their hands, they backed out of the door all apologies for waking us up! Later after breakfast, when we went to pay our bill, we learned that the General himself had taken in hand all our expenses. Trouble was brewing in Iran and we often wonder what became of him. Probably, after the fall of the Shah, he rejoined his daughters who were at school in Paris.

Another bus ride and we arrived at Isfahan, the fabulous city of flowers, carpets and rugs, with exceptionally beautiful architecture. During our twenty-four stay here, we took a taxi to the Holy Mountain of Fire – a place of powerful sacred energy – where I ruined a very smart pair of boots!

Beyond Isfahan and about 45 miles north-east of Shiraz, which suffered much from earthquakes in the nineteenth century, lies the main city of Persepolis. The building of Persepolis was commenced under Darius I (522–485 BC). Today it is one of the finest ancient ruins in the world, a magnificent visual experience, with its mountainous cliffs on one side forming dramatic, natural retaining walls. In juxtaposition to this superb ruin was a cluster of tents erected especially for a celebration to mark an event in the history of Persepolis. Kings and queens from all over the world were invited to attend this special function and each had individual living and sleeping quarters. In addition to this complex, there was an enormous, dominating 'big top' for receptions and banquets. The chandeliers were all of plastic and made in Italy (much to Joseph's annoyance). 'A complete lapse in taste,' he muttered. It struck us as farcical that a charge was made to visit the tents, whilst the ruins were free! Alas! Poor Darius; he must have turned in his grave.

Time to move on. Another hair-raising and uncomfortable night bus ride to the border town of Abadan, which we reached at the unearthly hour of 4 a.m. What can one do at 4 a.m.? Walk or take a cab, if you can find one. We found one and asked to be taken to Basra. No, sir! Relations were strained with Iraq and the taxi could only go as far as the Iranian side of no man's land – where we were unceremoniously dumped to face another military frontier teeming with soldiers. We would have to walk across no man's land: no transport whatsoever was available. A leering sentry, with rifle, pointed the direction. It was about five miles to the Iraqi frontier. Timidly we started to walk, giving casual glances behind our backs in case bullets started flying around. None did. It was now about 6 a.m. and the heat was already becoming intolerable.

This was not a walk in the charming countryside of England: it was a march across wasteland with no sign of life. The odd abandoned shed dominated the bleak landscape. When we reached the Iraqi side of no man's land, we were treated to a slightly kinder welcome and offered water. But when it came in an old enamel basin it did not look 'potable' so we satisfied our hosts by washing our hands and faces.

While awaiting the inspection of passports, I was sitting beside a Jordanian gentleman, who was travelling in a small car with all his family and luggage. With typical kindness, he took pity on us and offered us a lift to Basra, some miles away. We all squeezed, unbelievably, into the tiny vehicle and off we went. He dropped us at the river bank, where we crossed to

Basra on a precariously small boat, rowed by a little boy. At last we arrived at Shatt al-Arab hotel and airport, just outside Basra, where our first move was to join the ticket queue and get the last two seats on a small plane to Baghdad for the next morning. Now we were ready for a good English breakfast of bacon and eggs, with untold quantities of tea, to combat our dehydration. The hotel was in a nostalgic 1930s British colonial style, and our vast bedroom was sheer luxury. The gardens made a shady retreat for us tired travellers – the calm after the storm! We prepared for Baghdad, where we stopped two nights to say goodbye to all our dear friends and embarked on the long voyage home, mostly by bus.

The bus to Damascus in Syria was unusual. Described as an air-conditioned desert bus, Joseph called it a cigar-shaped phallic symbol: it gave the impression of speeding through the desert at 200 miles an hour, but in fact only succeeded in going rather slower than a normal bus! The interior resembled a poor man's Concorde and the air conditioning was defective. Attempts were made to correct it by pouring in chunks of ice. This failed miserably and only flooded the floor. So we all suffered till we arrived at the Iraq–Syrian border after midnight. Here a small shanty town described as a frontier 'port' possessed a toilet block for travellers, several WCs and a row of wash-hand basins. They had all been blocked and overrun for some time. This rest stop was called 'The Baghdad Cafe' but it was best to use the desert! Perhaps that was why it was described as a desert bus? Fortunately, I had learned in India never to travel without food and drink, so we dined on dates and nuts from Tehran, and a delicious whole chicken, cooked on the spit in Baghdad, and stuffed with rice and fruits.

Staying briefly in Damascus, where Joseph wanted to see the Great Mosque and I wanted to visit the house where St Paul was let down in a basket to escape his persecutors, we treated ourselves to a taxi and the intelligent driver gave us a history lesson. The journey through Lebanon was worth all the hardships. This small country, mountainous and beautiful, was a revelation. Not so the journey from Adana bus station to Ankara in Turkey. The bus on which we had reserved places was already full and double-booked, so we were transferred to a rather shabby vehicle as second best. Second best it proved to be.

In Europe the bus's bald tyres would never have been allowed on the road. The first tyre burst when the bus veered to avoid an elderly woman riding a donkey side-saddle. She landed on the side of the road, apparently unhurt. At least she was alive enough to curse us. The donkey disappeared over the edge and into the bushes. The bus did not stop. Shortly afterwards, another bald tyre burst. No doubt the driver and his sidekick blamed the old woman's curses. They transferred us to a different bus which was much safer, but already quite full. They managed to squeeze us all on board but many passengers, including us, had to stand in the aisle and I left behind a very precious scarf in that old wreck of a bus.

We were commandeered by Farouk, a charming young

Turkish army officer, who offered his seat. He spoke fluent English. We had got to know him quite well by the time we reached Ankara and he offered us his hospitality. We arrived at his apartment as his guests for the night. After turning out his flat-mate, he offered us the main bedroom. Breakfast in the morning consisted of a huge spread of hams, cheeses and sweetmeats. Farouk then insisted that as we were on our way to Istanbul, we should look up his parents: his father was a professor of English there.

He telephoned home to request his parents to prepare his room for us and when we arrived in Istanbul their welcome was very cordial. His mother and their three daughters, one of whom spoke English, were kind and hospitable. We visited the three mosques of the hill: Sancta Sophia, the oldest, going back to the fifth century, was especially haunting. Istanbul, with its many souks and with the Bosporus running through it, was fascinating and boisterous. Farouk's father invited us to join them for a cruise on the Black Sea but we were unable to accept. Time had run out. The next stop was Athens. We had pre-paid tickets to go by boat but there was no boat for ten days, so we opted regretfully for a quick flight there.

From Athens's port, Piraeus, we took the ferry to Brindisi in Italy. We had decided to work our way through Italy from south to north, with a detour to see Joseph's father. In Venice we took a small train for about 30 miles to Maniago in the Friuli part of the province of Veneto. This picturesque place lies at the foot of the Alps – a landscape of towering mountains, reaching 6,000 feet above sea level, with charming villages nestling at their feet. Maniago is the birthplace of the most delicious ice-cream in the world. When you have eaten it your taste buds have reached a never-to-be-forgotten climax!

Joseph's father was not expecting us travellers. He was over-joyed and, being the great romantic he was, serenaded us on his mandolin. We had a secret mission. Joseph's father had written during our last month in Baghdad, to say that a girl in nearby Fanna claimed her husband was an Iraqi and lived in Baghdad, and that he was the father of her son – would we look him up? We did look him up. We arranged to meet in the Baghdad Hotel. He was a bit suspicious of our enquiry, being indeed the father of her son but not prepared to take responsibility for them. I think the girl was only trying to establish her reputation as a decent married lady in her small community, and not an unmarried mother. I hope we cleared her name. It gave me the sense that the world is a very small place. The son, when we met him, was about seven years of age, handsome and the image of his father.

We travelled back to London in the hot summer of 1974, returning from Venice and Rome to the South of France to visit friends near the Bay of St Maxime. Then, it was our beloved Paris, the last stop before we took the train at the Gare du Nord for the journey to Victoria, London.

Our house in Wimbledon (which Joseph had bought in 1971) was welcoming and cosy. The weather was glorious and our roses in full bloom, but Great Britain was facing a major recession. While Joseph was struggling to re-establish himself in London, the American Hospital was calling for my return to Paris. It looked as if the tale of two cities must recommence. I began to look forward to a life in Paris with new responsibilities and new adventures. Of course I would miss Joseph but I knew he would soon be joining me there.

The search for a *pied-à-terre* began again, and this time we found an artist's studio, in the 5th *arrondissement*. This was on the fourth and top floor of a courtyard residence with enormous grilled gates. It contained two french windows, a working fireplace and a mezzanine, the whole being supported by fantastic beams. My friends and I used much elbow grease to restore the studio, which was situated in an enviable position near the Sorbonne and Notre Dame. Joseph returned to London and loved his regular visits to Paris. We were still very much individuals though deeply committed to each other. And together in Paris we painted the town red.

CHAPTER 10

ACUPUNCTURE TRAINING AND STUDY IN CHINA

Chinese medicine and pharmacology are a great treasure-house, and efforts should be made to explore them and raise them to a higher level. – Chairman Mao

It was during this period in Paris that I discovered acupuncture. I was nursing a prominent and dramatic woman whom we shall call Lucie, and who was admitted to the American Hospital with a broken ankle. A very popular lady, she had founded a theatre company in Paris and was surrounded by the artistic elite. A real beauty and *femme fatale*, one evening she gave me a periodical to read in which there was an interesting article about drug addiction and preventive medicine where acupuncture was mentioned. I suggested she should try acupuncture and as soon as her ankle was fit enough, I took her for a session. She was not patient with the treatment so the acupuncture could not work, but I wanted to experience this age-old science for myself.

I decided to have a consultation for a sinus problem. The condition cleared completely in two sessions and I felt light and free, as if walking on air. Later I learned that acupuncture releases endorphins into the bloodstream: these are morphine-like substances usually secreted by the pituitary gland. The freedom of finding and measuring the benefits of such an old science gave me much happiness. Ever since my childhood in Ireland I had searched for a form of healing that did not involve drugs. My mind and energy were stimulated and I knew that at last I had come to the end of a long search for an alternative to allopathic medicine: acupuncture.

Medical people today often have closed minds. Most doctors, nurses and other practitioners start off with an idealistic desire to help humanity but their training can stunt and blight their vision, by its emphasis on the rational and the materialistic. We have moved away from the ancient practice of observation: looking at people with our eyes and listening with a compassionate heart to the sound of their voices telling us of their complaints. (The tone of the voice is the surest of diagnostic tools.) We need not only scientific precision, but also spiritual depth to resonate with the being of the person needing help. With this we can diagnose, making prognoses and heal.

Illness frequently occurs to bring us to an awareness of ourselves and to a higher understanding of our destiny; it teaches us to look into ourselves and to take steps towards finding a cure. Through the experience we may become totally different human beings, and reach a spiritual transformation otherwise undreamed of. Healing is bringing oneself into harmony with the universe and the Divine creative force. It makes us whole and happy, and happiness is heaven.

Sadly, health practitioners are often too exhausted to heed

the promptings of the spirit. Their lives are filled with work, leaving no time or space for maintaining their own well-being. Work *is* a very important ingredient in the recipe of life. It keeps us healthy and stimulates our spirit – but the search for ultimate perfection must allow time for recreation too. It is a key to wholeness: literally, it re-creates us.

In France in 1979 I read an advertisement for students who wished to learn the ancient science of acupuncture with a Chinese doctor, Lily Chung, in London. I telephoned Dr Chung and after an interview was admitted to the study of this ancient art: my youthful dreams of China had begun to materialise! Although the Chinese language was the main barrier, we learned in English with a smattering of Chinese. After much study, we finally passed our exams and I enlisted with the rest of the group to go to Guangzhou in China for a postgraduate course at Zhongsan Medical College. This started on the 22nd of January 1981.

When I telephoned Joseph to tell him he was as usual full of enthusiasm; he would have come with me but his own architectural company was in its infancy. There were fifteen in our group, led by our teacher. On the flight out I met Dr Margaret MacDonald, who was destined later to play an important role in my life.

Once in Guangzhou, we spent the mornings observing acupuncture treatment in the outpatients department. As we were there for three weeks, we had time to see the changes that occurred in the various conditions treated.

Presenting symptoms were as varied as tinnitus and a haemorrhoid prolapsed rectum. We saw the symptoms of Bell's palsy greatly alleviated by needles applied to local points. Many of the patients were children. A ten-year-old was cured of bed-wetting while we were there. I particularly remember a four-year-old with hyperactivity, whose spasms were due, it appeared, to vaccinations in the USA. As soon as the acupuncture pins were inserted in his cranium and linked up to a mild electromagnetic machine, the child became calm and peaceful. His condition required much acupuncture, but I hope the results gave the child a better quality of life. On one occasion we witnessed an operation with acupuncture used as anaesthetic. It was unbelievable to see the patient participate fully in the procedure.

After outpatients, we would wander back through the gardens to our hotel for lunch. Dr Margaret MacDonald was an eye specialist who had 'seen the light' at the same time as myself: that if in our culture there was an awareness of emotional and spiritual health as well as the physical, illness and imbalance of energies would be detected before they reached an explosive point. Opting out of mainstream thinking, we believed that all medicine in the future would be preventive. We especially enjoyed each other's company, exploring together different faces of Chinese life. The young people were very cheerful and chatty. The old men practised their daily martial art exercise of t'ai chi, often hanging their pet bird's cage on the nearby branch of a tree while they did it. The gardens were full of beautiful chrysanthemums. Even the ceramic rubbish bins seemed to me like fabulous antique objects.

In 1981 t'ai chi was taken very seriously in China. In the 1950s when many doctors had either been killed or left the country, people waiting for medical attention had no option but to learn t'ai chi to support their health, to great effect. And it is not only in China that necessity turns us back to health therapies that have been known to work for millennia. One of these that we are apt to forget in the West is exercise. Exercise is vitally important to ensure good functioning of the lymphatic system, which relies on gravity and the natural pressures of muscles when you move your body weight. Yoga, Pilates and the Alexander Technique are excellent for toning our bodies. Breathing correctly with the abdominal muscles exchanges stale air for fresh and gets the ribcage and the diaphragm moving. This stimulates the oxygen supply to the brain and helps us understand how the smallest muscles need exercise, oxygen and movement. Keeping fit requires hard work and much discipline. You cannot expect an overnight transformation from a stressed life to one of peace and harmony. Like the Chinese, we must not be dismayed if it takes years to become a new person!

After our meal we went to the hospital for lectures (in English), many of which were about modern research and physiology. Others were about case histories, using the traditional approach and methods of diagnosis and treatment. To my great satisfaction, I learned that acupuncture and moxibustion (burning a herb on the patient's skin to restore harmony in the muscles) can be traced as far back as the Stone Age, when knives and other sharp-edged tools were invented to meet humans' needs. These instruments were used to relieve pain and disease and were known to the ancient Chinese as *Bian*.

In the Han Dynasty (206 BC–220 AD) there was a book called *Shio Weh Jie Zi* (Analytical Directory of Characters), a passage of which explains that *Bian* means using sharp stones on the acupuncture points to treat diseases. It may represent the most primitive acupuncture method of all, from neolithic times. The use of fire created conditions for the technique of moxibustion. The hot stones were replaced by needles made of bone or bamboo. In the Shang Dynasty, from *c.* 1200–800 BC, casting techniques were developed and it became possible to make bronze needles. The use of metal for needles was highly significant in the treatment since the conduction they produced while being used led to the discovery of the channels of energy which lace the body. All over China, the use of acupuncture developed rapidly and continued to the end of the Ching Dynasty (AD 1644–1912). However, the rulers of the Ching Dynasty despised the treatments for their simplicity and low cost, and went so far as to issue a decree banning their practice. But owing to the wide acceptance and belief in the therapy by the masses of labouring people, this art of healing survived. In Europe a Dr E. Kampfer introduced acupuncture to Germany in 1683. In 1863, when *The Medicine of China* was published in France, acupuncture and moxibustion were included in its contents. The practice of acupuncture was brought back to France in about 1929, the year of my birth, by Georges Soulie de Morant.

By a stroke of luck or destiny, Georges Soulie de Morant was able to study Mandarin from a very young age with a Chinese scholar who lived with friends of his family. Georges was educated by the Jesuits in Neuilly sur Seine. When the premature death of his father had forced him to renounce his passion to heal humanity and study medicine he opted for banking and was sent to China by the Banque Léhideux because of his fluency in Chinese. Soon he was engaged by the Minister of Foreign Affairs and nominated Consul de France in Shanghai and sent to Yunnan-Fou. During an outbreak of cholera, he noticed that the sick who were treated by acupuncture recovered faster than those treated by conventional medicine. This encouraged Georges to obtain a degree in Chinese Traditional Medicine, Art and Literature. He was acupuncture's ambassador to France. He suffered much, because his ideas met with fierce criticism. He died in Paris of a heart attack in 1955, aged seventy-seven.

While we were in China Madam Mao (Jiang Qing) was standing trial for treason. In 1974 Chairman Mao had regained Party command but in 1980 he was visibly ailing and his wife – known as the Dragon Lady – took over the leadership. Now she herself was tried and found guilty. Her gang of four had fallen from grace and we could detect an optimistic cheerfulness in the streets. Politics notwithstanding, our stay was a search for greater freedom in our own lives, and those of others, by the use of acupuncture needles (or, as I call them, 'pins'). At the end of our sojourn we sat for our final examination and came away with another certificate.

We had begun a new chapter in our journey – where would our compass point us?

In China, every other evening the students in our group had dinner together in a nearby restaurant. When we were on our own, Margaret and I wandered through the streets of Guangzhou which were teeming with bicycles. Young Chinese, hearing us speak, would stop and chat with us in excellent English. Margaret asked one of these young men, who spoke it exceptionally well, why he wasn't at university. 'It's too late, I'm a lorry driver,' he replied. 'I'm twenty-six years old.'

Sometimes we visited the huge department store reserved for tourists and helped the cheerful assistants with their English homework. They particularly liked our accents, preferring them to that of Americans.

Margaret and I would discuss all of this as we sipped Cointreau in my room. We were touched by the intelligence and friendliness of a people living very frugal lives. Professor Wu Xinjin, who organised the course, lived in a three-bedroomed flat with her in-laws and her son and his wife. She spoke fluent French, German and English and had degrees in physiology, Western medicine and traditional Chinese medicine. I do not think Professor Wu Xinjin would abandon her country and people for the material riches of the West, as so many economic migrants have done.

To a very intelligent guide we had, Margaret voiced her shame that many people in England at that time thought the Cultural Revolution a good idea. It would be a lesson for academics to learn about life in rural villages, she said.

'Yes,' he said. 'It would have been a good idea if it had been for a year. My parents were away for ten years. Because the village paid the university costs, they chose their own people not me, so I didn't get to university.'

Several things did impress us about Mao's legacy. The men on the course were told that one could not buy sex in China. Gambling was forbidden – though we did see the occasional game of Mah Jong being played quietly in the streets, while observers looked out for police. We saw people who enjoyed working together, hand painting in ceramics factories and weaving in silk factories, although the conditions were primitive.

On our last day, Margaret and I went to purchase a scroll painting each in a very small shop. People came in off the street to watch us. Margaret chose a cockerel, to the great thrill of cheers – it was the year of the cockerel, which we had not realised. I chose a beautiful, fat frog climbing a banana tree. This choice was also approved, the frog being the symbol of France for me – and of good fortune, of course!

We left Canton with immense gratitude, having been among

the first foreigners to be allowed into China after the Cultural Revolution. One of the most important things we had learned was the value of taking responsibility for our own health and not relying on other people. We must learn how our bodies are put together, how organs function and what improves or helps the body maintain equilibrium. In my opinion, nutrition, from the time the baby is in the womb and thereafter, is supremely important. If we look at animal and plant life, we can learn enormous lessons from the way they take what nutrients they need from the best source, a healthy earth, one hopefully not polluted by man.

Another thing we learned in China was that argil, or clay, is a valuable source of minerals. It is widely used in France, and in fact throughout the world, in the shape of remedies, poultices, beauty products and as nourishment. Did not Christ take the clay and mix His own saliva with it to anoint and heal the man born blind? The curative properties of argil are recognised by scientists, but still not accepted by allopathic doctors. It is used for the extraordinary power of its radioactivity, naturally balanced by the Earth, and its capacity to vitalise and heal a sick organ. Argil is the angel of health and, according to the Chinese, consists of the five elements essential to conduct a cure: air, fire, water, wood and metal. The Earth is a fruitful mother. The Sun gives light and energy to the solar system and the Earth absorbs the different forces of air, water and sunlight to germinate and bring fruits and plants to term. Life in all its beauty. In ancient times the Chinese, Indians, Turks, Egyptians and South Americans used argil in external and internal remedies. In our own times Gandhi was an ardent supporter of natural medicines, in particular the use of clay.

The Earth, our mother, is giving us through her therapeutic properties another chance to heal ourselves. Chemically the Earth contains the principal salts in the correct balance needed by humans. Bones are two-thirds mineral, and the best remedy for bone maintenance is the use of clay. Its magnesium content is especially beneficial in fighting cancer. Calcium is sovereign in preventing osteoporosis, anaemia and tuberculosis.

The Western way is to dominate, humiliate and even eradicate any way of life that gets in the way of our kind of 'progress' – a man-made progress invented scarcely a few centuries ago. Having assumed superiority, it becomes more than acceptable for us to bulldoze nature, native societies and thousands of years of civilisation. Primitive people used herbs and earth cures without knowing analytically how or why they cured: they simply observed, accepted and believed their own eyes. Today we live in a world where we feel we must have scientific proof – yet how often we are let down. Acupuncture, moxibustion treatment and the use of herbs, for example, are still kept at arm's length by the majority of the medical profession. They have forgotten that health comes partly through contentment; from cultivating an inner peace and making time for leisure and sleep. The big killer in today's society is stress brought about by pressures of work – and lack of love. We sink into a decline and the tree of life becomes blighted.

I returned from China to Paris and worked for a couple of years in liaison with a doctor who sent me patients requiring natural therapy (acupuncture, herbs and other drug-free methods). My dream was to start a healing centre – to change the world. I was to learn there is only one person I was given to change – and that is myself. I was to face my greatest trial, my anger, my resignation, my growth – my cure. The most difficult aspect of the illness ahead of me was the powerlessness of always being in someone else's hands. My faith had to be tested. I was my own guinea pig; the years in isolation due to illness were passed in prayer and study of all kinds – like Job on his dunghill.

I was to learn that health is also having *faith* in the higher aspects of human nature. Health is having *hope*, because without hope there is no life. Health is *love* of our selves and others.

In truth, love is the life blood of faith and hope and together they create a healthy body, mind and spirit: the Trinity of our being.

CHAPTER 11

SERIOUS ILLNESS

*Zero is where all real fun starts because there is too
much counting everywhere else.* – Hafiz

In the spring of 1983 – having no idea how things were to
change only a few months later – Joseph and I spent a restora-
tive week exploring Sicily on holiday.

On Volcano Island we applied sulphur mud to our bodies
and washed in the warm sea-water. We thanked God that some
of the great things in life were still free. Afterwards we left Sicily
renewed and detoxed, but the week had passed too quickly.
When we returned to London, I decided it was time to put
down my roots with Joseph in Nevern Square, where we now
had a flat, and establish my acupuncture practice in England.
At that time London was still firmly closed to the wider vision
of preventive medicine. Introducing myself and my new-found
ideas was harder than climbing the highest mountain.
Acupuncture was seen as useful only for people who wanted to
stop smoking. I was dismayed: I wanted to tell the whole world
about this great natural means of curing or preventing disease.
So I booked a stand at the very first Body, Mind and Spirit
Festival and slowly clients came. I built a small practice mainly
through word of mouth. I continued to study other fields of
energy such as magnetism, and the Alexander Technique with

a wonderful teacher, Jean Robinson. Both of these methods were of enormous benefit to me personally.

My old intestinal problem from my convent days suddenly recurred. At the start of my new life in London I found I was reminded of my mortality and my break with India. Various tests which my GP advised proved negative, but the symptoms persisted so a colonoscopy was arranged. This test was carried out by a surgeon in the London Clinic. He was so busy chatting and laughing with his two assistants, he forgot to unscrew the instrument to release the air he had injected to inflate the intestine. When I was wheeled back to the recovery room my abdomen was huge – like an eight-month pregnancy. The pain was so acute, I rang the bell for assistance. The nurse came and I asked how I was going to get rid of the air. Curtly she replied, 'Get rid of it naturally.' Joseph was at work, so I took a taxi home. I just managed to get through the door before I had a heavy haemorrhage.

My confidence had not been boosted by the dismissive way in which I had been treated and I decided to have recourse to natural therapies (Chinese herbs, acupuncture and good diet). After Christmas, Joseph insisted on taking me back to Autun in France to consult Dr Cusson, who knew best my medical history. He examined the X-rays and advised surgery, explaining that the condition was contained and that there was nothing to fear – the operation would be straightforward. On our return we stopped in Paris for me to have a screening test, which was arranged by one of my Parisian colleagues. The bleeding polyp showed up, unquestionably malignant, but there were no secondaries. The blood picture was excellent.

Back in London, I saw a wonderful surgeon and was admitted to King's College Hospital for further investigations. The whole business was a nightmare. The hygiene standards were appalling; the nursing – mainly by agency nurses – was unbelievably poor. The only great human beings there were the surgeon and the sister-in-charge. While I myself worked in the nursing profession, in Ireland, India, England or France I had never been confronted with standards of basic cleanliness as low as these. Sinks were dirty, the floor was filthy and rubbish in bags sat in the corridors. There was no sense of the safety of being in a clean, freshly made bed while being cared for with human compassion. I asked for cleaning materials and did what I could. The years of 1983 and 1984 were spent trying to reduce the polyp and heal myself with the means at my disposal, but Western medicine had more lessons to teach me.

Appalled with the state of the Health Service and hospitals in London, I decided, after much persuasion on the part of my Parisian colleague, to opt for treatment in Paris. I was recommended another surgeon of high repute, who worked in the Clinique d'Alleray. The operation was done under spinal anaesthesia, so I heard everything that went on – even the surgeon speaking to his wife on the telephone. Surgery was scheduled for 10 a.m. but took place at 6.30 p.m. and lasted for two and a half hours. It was not a smooth procedure. The intestinal cleansing, essential preparation for surgery, was of a poor standard and quite inadequate. The medical report of the operation confirms that my own condition was excellent and everything augured well. In the surgeon's judgement it was not necessary to insert a drainage tube at the site of the anastomosis (where the two ends of the intestine were sutured together). In fact, this tube is essential to remove toxins from the site and is standard practice even in less serious abdominal operations. What were they thinking of?

The morning following the operation I began to experience a pain like razor blades cutting into me. By now the surgeon had flown off to operate on another patient in the Middle East and left me in the care of the anaesthetist, who happened to be his own brother. My body became more and more toxic. I was in great pain. I experienced frightening rigors as the poisons built up in my body. When I asked for help I was told to take a deep breath. Of course Joseph rushed from London to be with me and was the only one to recognise the danger I was in, but he never, even by a suggestion, exposed his own personal fears or heartbreak. A week after the operation I was discharged into the care of my friend, Geneviève, in this condition. Three weeks later I was back on the operating table having surgery to save my life.

I returned to London with a nurse, by wheelchair and ambulance. Halfway to Charles de Gaulle Airport the ambulance crew stopped and demanded to be paid 500 francs: we would be left on the roadside if we could not produce the money, they said. On a stretcher and unable to write, I had no strength to be angry. My nurse wrote the cheque and I signed it. At the airport we found that a strike meant an unlimited delay to our flight. The nurse phoned Joseph to put him in the picture. But finally we made it home, where Joseph was waiting to carry me upstairs. He nursed me with such love. I did not want to die because I could not bear to be parted from him.

Each day brought new problems, which I do not want to dwell on. At last, I returned to see a wonderful English surgeon, Mr Dawson, who took me on in spite of everything. He did not hold out much hope of recovery but his advice was, 'You must eat liver, and salad of endive and fish even if you are not hungry.' Joseph found Ming, a wonderful Chinese lady, to nurse me when he was at work. Ming completely took charge of me and the house, shopping, cooking and cleaning. She nursed me back to health in the traditional Chinese fashion with herbs and love. I learned a vast amount from her – and what a great woman she was. Here was one my father would have called 'an angel with crushed wings' who flew to my rescue. She cooked me bird's nest, a Chinese cure – ginseng and poached fish. Without her, I'm sure I could not have survived. In looking after me she also looked after Joseph. Her presence was like radiant sunshine.

I called upon my old friend Margaret MacDonald, who came immediately. Years later she told me that on seeing me in the bed her first impression was that I wouldn't make it. Margaret gave me acupuncture: when she left I knew my channels were opened and I would recover. The pins, together with all the other tender loving care, would do it. She came once a week. Joseph was the only one who truly saw my pain. He used to lie beside me on the bed and hold my hand with concern and tenderness but we had to sleep in different rooms because I did not want my restlessness to disturb him.

The nuns at Roehampton Convent took care of the linen and laundry. I was surrounded by loving and sympathetic friends who in time I came to look on as daughters; and there was the occasional son, like Alahn MacRae, who would come and sit by my bed and just hold my hand in silence.

At the end of 1985, though still struggling, Joseph and I held a joyful 'Musical Evening' to give thanks to God for giving me back my life. My old friend and spiritual mentor, Monsignor Patrick Keaveny, said a special Mass in the house. Ming and I had cooked a supper of fresh wild salmon. Our Norwegian friend, Sonja Nerdrum, came and gave forth with her dramatic voice as well as bringing a home-made salad in a huge Victorian basin. Joseph sang the *Merry Widow* duet with Sandra Ford, a great friend of ours and an opera singer with the sweetest voice. They waltzed together. The accompanist Valda Plucknett played the piano. Later Joseph sang Neapolitan folk songs, and my own favourite Irish air 'She moved through the Fair' was sung by Sandra Ford. Sonja sang fiery and dramatic songs from *Aida* and *Carmen*.

For several years I suffered from toxaemia. Little by little I regained strength. Throughout, my biggest blessing was that I never lost interest in life and I wanted to get better for Joseph. A great part of the cure was his insistence on taking me to Covent Garden so that we could listen to our favourite operas together. Painfully I climbed up those stairs to the gods to drink in the music. The biggest sacrifice was having a colostomy. I had two operations in 1985, but toxaemia prevented the removal of the rabbit warren of abscesses still left behind. Only in 1988 was Mr Dawson finally able to operate and remove the root cause. In November of that year the colostomy was closed and I was given back a poor battered body with the recommendation that I have a check-up every six months. I was fifty-nine and my hair had turned very grey, but Joseph was beside me and I knew his love would see me through.

During the hard uphill climb to recovery I could not work. I was being looked after. But I was learning in the school of suffering, especially the lessons of humility, dependence and the importance of learning to receive as well as to give. After a while the occasional person came to me for acupuncture, drawn by personal introduction in that strange way through which people of feeling find and recognise each other. I learned to empathise with the energy field of sensitive people, and about the compassion between healer and patient. I told no one about my own personal health problems.

One of those who found me was Maureen Doherty who came to me with an eye problem. Specialists in Paris and London with one voice had told her that she would have to take cortisone for the rest of her life and wear a patch over her eye. She was just thirty-three.

Apparently the first acupuncture pin which I inserted in her hand connected with her eye channel and Maureen's pain disappeared. She didn't tell me straight away in case the pain returned, but that afternoon I received the most wonderful box full of lily of the valley. It was the month of May and the French always celebrate with these flowers, a very old custom supposed to bring you luck. Maureen had also lived and loved in Paris; an artist and visionary, she became a great friend in the years that followed. Later she told me that the first time I opened the door to her, she looked at my face and said to herself: *This is the face of a monk or a nun.* Then she followed me up the stairs and saw the black lace stockings I was wearing and thought: *She is one of us, after all.* Maureen at that time did the PR for the designer Issey Miyake. It was she who asked if I would consider being photographed by Snowdon. She explained that Issey Miyake did not use professional models but had his designs photographed on men and women 'of character'. I felt honoured. I wore his clothes for the 1987–88 Portfolio, photographed by Lord Snowdon and in the company of the singer-songwriter Joan Armatrading, the sculptor Elizabeth Frink, the Indian fashion designer and sociologist Asha Sarabhai, Joanne Brogden, Head of Fashion at the Royal College of Art, Liliane Lijn, the visual artist, and the industrial designer and patron Jeremy Fry.

CHAPTER 12

HRH THE PRINCESS OF WALES

The Pearl
Scientists agree that a pearl is the product of pain.
The oyster lies in its bed at the bottom of the ocean,
it is invaded by a tiny parasite which succeeds in
getting into the very heart of the oyster. All the healing
resources rush to the site of the wound to bring about
healing – the scar or healed wound becomes a pearl.
Where there are no wounded oysters there are no
pearls! – Anon

On the 5th of September 1989 I had a telephone call from Princess Diana, asking me if I would visit her. A mutual friend, Mara Berni, had told Diana about me, and that I was working as a healer. Next morning I took a green taxi to Kensington Palace and met the Princess, who was waiting for me in her dressing gown and bare feet. She was suffering physically, emotionally and spiritually. Her hands and feet were blue and she presented a very tormented landscape. Diana was very fragile, very low in energy and in extreme need of affection. Her two boys were jewels.

Diana had felt rejected from a tender age. She was angry. She had so much love and compassion in her heart and it seemed only her children were capable of recognising it. She was a child at heart: her first impulse was to please others. Later, this was to get her into difficulty. But her love was limitless and boundless and she had no one to receive or give her love in the measure she needed to give and receive. The caring role satisfied her need only in part. She herself needed nurturing, spiritual guidance and love.

Diana was innocent of the world she was thrown into, she had no preparation, she was not at ease and never really relaxed. We grow wise by stages and sometimes a whole lifetime is necessary to gain wisdom. Diana had an open heart and arms outstretched to help those in need. The public have been well informed over the years about the various aspects of her personality and activities but what I perceived was that the eyes that saw Diana were incapable of recognising her essence. The essence of Diana was spiritual. She was a very old soul dressed in modern garb come back to teach us about love.

I took the Princess's medical history, balanced her chakras and introduced her to my combination of treatments. After about two weeks I shared with her a secret of my own: that I had spent twenty years in a convent and because of ill health finally had to ask His Holiness, Pope Paul VI, to leave the life of serving God 'in His poor'. This confession of mine was the spiritual foundation on which our friendship was built. I gave her many many books, among them *The Imitation of Christ*. She was so grateful for the slightest gift and after her verbal thanks, a letter always followed.

For almost six and a half years I saw Princess Diana weekly.

I advised her to be patient, not to store up bitterness in her heart and guided her to study the different religions, introducing her to the philosophy of a spiritual teacher – Omraam Mikhael Aivanhov. I encouraged her to be herself, to follow the voice of her heart, to help the helpless, to mould her life on the life of Christ. Christ urges us to place our own light like a lighted candle in a candlestick where all may see it.

Visualisation and meditation require no physical output, but the spiritual benefits are incalculable. The Princess made good progress and learned fast. I foresaw a spiritual mission for her from my very first visit.

Soon it became apparent that marriage counselling was not appropriate. Princess Diana often said she had great difficulty holding together relationships and friends. Even those who sincerely wanted to help her were cut off. I can understand her dilemma. The world sometimes seems very tired. Disillusion and discouragement cause fatigue (a Tower of Babel). People draw their main source of energy from their psychic natures. Happiness comes from within the soul. Diana was not happy. The gradual decline in creative self-expression is a sure symptom of deep-seated problems.

As Princess Diana's spiritual life grew stronger, her physical well-being also improved. She was not deranged, far from it – just dying of thirst. She was as quick as lightning and seized every opportunity to make up for her poor results at school by learning about real life in the real world. She asked a lot of questions about medical conditions she did not understand.

After Prince William was born, Diana suffered from post-natal depression, and again after Prince Harry's birth. When I last met her there was still evidence that she had not completely recovered. Some women never get over postnatal depression. I had known a very sad case in France where a mother who had just one female child was scarred for life by postnatal trauma in spite of having a loving husband. In my experience this condition is not well understood. If only the union of the child and the mother could be blissful for the first six weeks and echo the happiness of the two people who conceive and have the child. In reality this time is often hell. The sudden dip in hormones throws the body's equilibrium out of balance. Often this is misinterpreted as a demand for attention, when in reality there is a great need for sweetness. Six weeks is the minimum recovery time a new mother needs. Without a supportive and understanding environment lifelong traumas can result, leading to resentment and even hatred.

Diana was constantly searching for love, for appreciation. She could not focus her life without love, and her capacity for it was enormous. When her two boys went away to school she was lonely and forlorn, returning to the palace alone. There was no partner to share the joys or sorrows of the day with, no arms to reach out and embrace her. Diana's judgement was impaired by this isolation. She had her flings and believed often in the wrong people. What a waste! Diana's great potential was ultimately poisoned because of the unfulfilled relationship with her husband, whom she loved: she was like a rudderless barque in a tempestuous sea. The hot pursuit of the media added to the torture.

During Princess Diana's visit to Calcutta in 1991 she wrote in a letter to me:

> I picked up a little boy who was blind and deaf. I hugged him so tightly hoping he could feel my love and healing coming through. I gazed at this alarmingly large number of children who were without parental love and was somewhat reassured by the care the Sisters were showing. After an hour there, I was taken to the Mother's Hospice for the Dying and there was the greatest impact . . . hundreds of beds lined the room with such sick men and women. Some crying, some sleeping and some dying – dying with dignity and with a carer beside them. I knew the individual was happy to be leaving this place under Mother Teresa's roof – probably the first time in their lives that someone had cared for them . . .
>
> The emotions running through the Hospice were very strong and the effect it had on me was how much I wanted and longed to be part of all this on a global scale.

All these aspirations were the voices from within, spurring Diana on – and thank God she enjoyed those spiritual flights while the paparazzi and media were recording what their poor blind eyes were seeing. Again we hear the voice of the Pharisees – accusing Diana of exhibitionism, vanity and playing to the camera. It is not easy to care for the sick, the infected and the dying and it requires real valour, real generosity, forgetfulness of self. Diana was born with Divine gifts which no amount of learning can impart. She was her own person, strong and witty. Her spiritual life was very private and she got her strength from prayer and spiritual reading. Flowers gave her immense happiness; her favourites were white freesias, roses and lilies. She had a particular distaste for orchids of any shape or colour, which must have been a personal association (not a happy one). The last armful of orchids was received on her last holiday, days before that fatal crash.

Princess Diana could not bear the 'kiss and tell, the cut and paste rogues' and took her revenge. The tabloids spread false reports, reaping vast amounts of money and poisoning people's lives. But she kept going despite the press. In secret she wept, but her smile and outstretched hands were ever ready to comfort those in need.

Touch is still the truest medium of expression. Hands are so important, they tell us much about a person. When two people shake hands, for example, they connect together a myriad chakra prints in their palms, which is why a friendly, heartfelt handshake can be a very uplifting healing experience. Diana could feel this energy in her hands and her touch linked with her own heart, and those of others. She couldn't help but take people in her arms.

In 1992, when the separation from Prince Charles was announced, Diana was desolate; and when the Anglican Church excluded her from their prayers she was devastated, seeking refuge in helping others to heal.

Diana's compassion was genuine. I know that from first-hand experience of it, when facing Joseph's heart operation in August 1995. Earlier that month, Princess Diana had invited Joseph and myself to lunch. She was a superb hostess. After a delicious meal and while we were still at table, Joseph asked if he could sing a song for her. On receiving an 'Of course, Joseph, please,' he sang 'Silent Worship' by Handel and later 'La Paloma' (The Dove).

When he had finished Diana said, 'Joseph, no one has ever sung for me like this at my table. I could hear your heart beating. You sing with such soul.'

This is the letter I wrote on the 21st of August to that graceful human being:

Dearest Princess Diana,

Thank you for a most delicious lunch on August 14th.

'The heart has its reasons,' to quote the Duchess of Windsor, and Joseph's heart was consoled to have your hands touch it – will the press get hold of this new conquest?

Healing hands, loving hearts mend the broken heart of the Universe.

Love is being in harmony with one and all – Give and Forgive!

United in that Big Heart we say thanks and may God keep you in the palm of His Hand.

Love and prayers.

Always, Joseph and Oonagh Toffolo

On the 31st of August 1995 Joseph was operated on by Professor Sir Magdi Yacoub, assisted by Mr Hasnat Khan, for a triple bypass and valvular repair. Twenty minutes after he arrived in intensive care, the Chinese nurse in charge noticed the drainage jars were full of blood. Joseph was having a massive haemorrhage. The cardiac arrest alarm pealed out its sinister message. Professor Yacoub had his scalpel in his hand, poised to operate on the next patient. He and the team rushed to Joseph's bedside and opened the chest wall. The bleeding was arrested and the heart restarted.

I was at home, waiting for a call to say surgery was completed. None came, but at the moment of the crisis, I had a huge pain in my heart. Thank God an old friend, Sister Mairead, was with me.

Quickly she got hold of the phone. Sister Mairead dialled. I was transfixed, unable to move. The person who took the call asked us to come immediately. Someone from the hospital had been trying to get in touch but had dialled the wrong digit. I blew out the candles and closed doors. We snatched our coats and ran out.

At the hospital pandemonium reigned. The sister-in-charge was quite beside herself. We were put in a small waiting room – we prayed – suddenly a nurse came in. 'Are you Mrs Zoffolo or something of that sound?' She took me into a ward full of men: there was no Joseph Toffolo. What was going to go wrong next? What were they doing with my beloved Joseph? Finally, a very nice anaesthetist came with his assistant and told us what had happened, the critical state Joseph was in – and would I stay the night?

Later we were able to see Joseph in the Intensive Care Unit.

He looked like death. I was allowed to sit by him and come and go as I pleased. That night I lay in the room previously assigned to Joseph, number 125. Sleep would not come, so I made several phone calls and then went to keep watch beside him in Intensive Care. I had phoned Princess Diana about 9 p.m. to put her in the picture. She told me she would have liked to come at once but her boys were at home so she would have to come in the morning. Next day she came at about 10 a.m. I was waiting for her and we had hardly spent five minutes together, when Mr Khan and his assistant came in. I introduced the Princess.

Joseph's condition was very serious. The bleeding was still oozing from somewhere. Mr Khan wanted my permission to take him back to the theatre to do an A–Z check on him. I looked at the intense and kind face of this man, whom I had seen so many times during the night. I took his hand and kissed it and said, 'Please look after him. He is very precious to us!' Mr Khan promised to come and give me a full report in room 125, as soon as he had finished operating. Princess Diana took me there, and made me lie down. She ordered scrambled egg and tea for me, while she herself took coffee. Joseph survived the third opening of the chest. Apparently the haemorrhage was caused by faulty clips which had gone undetected and Mr Khan had to replace them with old-fashioned suturing.

As Joseph recovered, he claimed that Mr Khan had a genius for making people feel good. I saw him as a kind and devoted surgeon, married to his profession – his calling. He was so good to us, even before the Princess appeared on the scene. Princess Diana came every day to see Joseph. Her visits were a real morale boost to us. The doctors, nurses and staff were all edified by her presence. When Joseph regained consciousness he had a succession of beautiful young women taking turns at his bedside 'The daughters' who had cared for me a few years earlier were now showering attention on Joseph. He likened himself to Wotan in *Die Walküre* with his seven daughters. Diana regularly took Joseph for walks in the corridor, bringing a smile to his face with her witty remarks, her love and unparalleled devotion.

However, very soon I started to receive cards and flowers from journalists, which caused me great distress. I told the hospital press office I did not want to give any statements or receive flowers. My chief concern was to protect Diana and to keep her out of the news, but of course that was not possible for long. Joseph did not suffer fools gladly and he complained to me that his bedroom was often a playground of visitors and that it disturbed his peace and tranquillity. Silence is an absolute necessity in healing sick patients and Joseph's recovery was greatly hampered by the lack of it. The paparazzi were on the prowl day and night. In the end they made our lives infernal. Later they used every conceivable intrigue to gain entrance to our home.

Princess Diana became very interested in heart surgery and asked me if I could get permission for her to attend an operation so she could promote the cause of such surgery for children. I was able to arrange for that wish to be granted. She paid great attention to learning as much as she could about illness and its causes. She used her intelligence. The Sunday morning Joseph left the hospital, Diana was there to see us off. Her compassion for the sick and the dying had a boundless power, which I am sure healed many scarred souls.

At Joseph's homecoming, we discovered our telephone was being tapped and although we were ex-directory, we were plagued by phone calls day and night. Journalists were constantly trying to gain entrance, blighting our lives. Laurence Tucker, our neighbour, tried hard to protect us and often ejected them from the house. But one intruder gained entrance under false pretences and wrote the most horrible and malicious article which made it sound as if we had gone to the press, which was quite untrue. I was especially devastated because it was just before Christmas, the season of goodwill. Joseph was still fragile. Diana was very upset and offended. Princess Diana needed the help of the media to promote her charitable and humanitarian efforts. She was affected by the media's, often untrue, reports and sometimes cut herself off from the very people who were faithful to her. I wrote to her and tried to explain, but received no answer. We changed our telephone number and I took refuge in silence. Joseph was very badly affected and it delayed his recovery, while my own health was again undermined.

I stopped seeing patients. I nursed Joseph through his slow return to health. We both needed seclusion to heal ourselves and I returned to my writings and my study.

Christ in his teachings said: 'You cannot serve two masters.' There is only real joy to be found in the infinite source and essence of Love, that is Christ. If we see nothing but Him, know no one but Him and hear nothing but Him, then we have reached infinite delights. But if we are caught in seeking the approval of others we are wrestling with a finite, mortal and fickle element. If we get ourselves entangled in what others do and say and think, we lose our own identity. We lose our way. When Princess Diana was in the company of the sick and the dying and away from 'the others', she was in touch with her real self – her atman, the Divinity within her. She was at ease with herself.

Diana and I had an unusual friendship: we were united in a common search for truth. For both of us, the goal was the healing of and caring for humanity, especially mothers and babies. It was a spiritual quest – a destiny. I had given Diana a set of Rosary beads during the first months of our getting to know each other; she was overjoyed and with hand on her heart promised to keep it with her for the rest of her life. We did not know how short that precious life was to be. I was told that on her deathbed in Paris the Rosary beads were found in her handbag and entwined between her fingers, and that the hospital chaplain anointed her.

For myself, I shall always remember Princess Diana in her own words, those she wrote to me in 1992:

I have a deep feeling of mission to be fulfilled. It has set me apart from others for a long time now. I had my questions answered in

Calcutta and I wish that it was possible to put my true feelings on to paper; but they run too deep and would frighten those around me with their intensity. I have an enormous amount inside me that I want to share with those who suffer or those who require light in their dark existences. The power comes from within and having responsibility gives us the power to make changes in our lives – maybe it is time!

Amen.

CHAPTER 13

REFLECTIONS ON DEATH

Grief is a dying within me, a great emptiness, a frightening void. – Cardinal Basil Hume

When sudden death claims our loved ones we think what a tragedy, what a waste. The pain of grief can hardly be endured. In the days and weeks following the sudden and horrible death of Diana the whole world, it seemed, woke up, and those who loved her felt their hearts pierced. The tragedy in Paris made those who did not love her strike their breasts: *mea culpa*. A silent hush descended on London. Everybody shared a special memory of Diana and could identify their lives with hers in some way. I believe her destiny was to open the heart chakra of the world. This gift involved suffering and pain. In her short life she did much to help humanity and brought about great changes in the House of Windsor.

She was a free spirit and did not fit into the royal mould, but she did love Charles. When that river of love was not used she turned to children, old people and humanity at large. Princess Diana was denied the ambassadorial role she wanted while on Earth but now, away from the cameras and empowered by a spiritual strength, her influence will never die. I am certain that her sons feel her presence and that eventually the scales of blindness will fall from the eyes of those who do not want to believe in God's love.

Princess Diana's light was shining too brightly for the myopic world we live in. Her dreams could only be realised and reach fruition in a more mature and enlightened society. Every time she thought she was understood and loved, the cameras and the media gave their ugly version of events, rupturing the good links that surrounded her and exposing her to fits of despair. Diana was frequently heard to say, 'When will I see the light at the end of the tunnel?' To me she said, 'Oonagh, if anything should happen to me would you please tell the world who I really was and not the person they made me out to be.'

Princess Diana was a chosen soul, full to the brim with love. She found no other vessel big enough to hold the contents of her own love. It had to flow out in other directions. Christ said simply, 'by their works ye shall know my disciples; judge not that ye be not judged.' Princess Diana no longer needs people to defend her, as there are neither titles nor icons in Heaven. How many people think of praying for Diana? How many people think about her new journey? The soul in spirit is not engaged in blissful adoration before the throne of God; life in the spirit is a continuation of life in our world. The work of purification continues but in an atmosphere of total love and light.

In a dream one night I saw Princess Diana arrive in the ante chambers of Paradise. There was great joy and immense sorrow at the tragedy. The music we heard at her funeral was an echo of the great chorus of alleluias of her reception in Heaven. The energy she brought over was like a blaze of music. The little children thronged about Diana and there was much laughter and many hugs; her father showed himself as a young man and she did not recognise him at first. What a meeting they had, a loving tête-à-tête where everything was forgiven and forgotten.

The Spencer family had already made a huge spiritual contribution to the Christian world. Princess Diana's great-uncle, the Anglican priest and scholar Ignatius Spencer, was one of the Victorian heroes who fought to create unity and common ground between the Christian Churches. He converted to Roman Catholicism and became a Passionist priest who actively promoted the movement of prayer for universal Christian unity in Great Britain and Europe. In his day he was thought to be either a prophet or a madman.

I gave Diana a little brochure, *Ignatius Spencer, Apostle of Christian Unity* (Catholic Truth Society Publications) which introduced her to her uncle. She had never heard of him! Diana wanted more than anything else in the world to spread love, but the language of love is not understood by everybody. The grief the world expressed was linked in people's minds with youth, beauty and life wasted, but Diana's life was not wasted and we should follow her in her dreams of helping the helpless, loving the unloved.

The secret of unhappiness is trying to please everybody: it is a moral impossibility and leads to compromise of our true selves. Many of us are influenced by the judgement of others, preoccupied with how others see us and speak about us. This leads to a restless spirit. When we begin to look inwards we discover our true selves. Diana did not feel at home with the high and mighty, she became completely disenchanted. She felt at ease with the sick and the humble of heart, like the little children who expected nothing from her but tender embraces – I call her the children's princess. Only God, the real essence of love, could fill her soul with happiness.

Alas! absence leads to forgetfulness, but let us not forget Diana's magnetism and love. She helped to tear away the stigma of AIDS, she befriended the lepers and supported the dying in Mother Teresa's hospice in Calcutta, and she publicised the issue of landmines, among many other causes. The real Diana has been lost in the whirlpool of many stories, books and films . . . yet she will remain a shining soul with feet of clay. For those who can, let them see the greatness of the love that was within her. Hopefully, one day Diana's memory will once again flourish and her wishes will be realised for the world she strove to change – and for which she shed so many tears . . .

When I began to write this chapter of the book, Joseph was by my side helping me with my story. On 18th March 1999 I awoke with a sense of foreboding and threw myself on my knees before the Madonna asking her to protect us because I knew something terrible was going to happen.

Joseph brought me my morning cup of coffee and at that moment our friend Sandra Ford phoned and asked how we were. I told her Joseph was by my side and that he looked so beautiful and so young and that he sent his love. She replied, 'We are not worried about Joseph any more; we are worried about you.'

I had promised a young man with cancer of the brain that I would visit him at eleven o'clock and Joseph insisted on taking me there. At parting I kissed Joseph's hand, said I love you and confirmed that we would meet for lunch at midday. I stood in the middle of the road waving until the car went out of sight. My visit took longer than I expected and I returned home at one o'clock. The car was not outside and I felt a physical pain in my heart. Words cannot tell my distress – my hopelessness. I phoned a friend, Katharine Warriner, to tell her of my premonition and with a gentle voice she tried to reassure me and told me to make myself a cup of tea. I was just pouring it when I heard a tapping at the door.

The messenger who brought the news was a young, most gentle and diplomatic policeman dressed in civilian clothes. I will always remember PC Richard Manning. He took me in his arms and told me that Joseph had died suddenly from a post-operative complication. At my request, he took me to the place where Joseph had died and then on to the Chelsea & Westminster Hospital to say farewell to the man who had loved and protected me. I looked at his handsome face and covered him with kisses, while tears flowed freely. Joseph had taught me many wonderful lessons about living life to the full, travelling, climbing mountains; about architecture and ancient civilisations. Even on the day he died he was organising his next major expedition.

Joseph's passion was music and opera. At his funeral service his friends, professional operatic singers and musicians from the Music Evenings which he had initiated in 1985, played the most sacred music and sang solos from Joseph's repertoire.

Two tributes in particular stand out. One from his friend, Robert Warriner:

> Joseph was a gifted artist and could draw very well. His understanding of space and perspective were no doubt put to good use in his practice as an architect. But Joseph's great love was music and being involved with it, especially opera and singing. He was always ready to give forth and sang for his friends at evening soirées. The most recent occasion was during Oonagh and Joseph's holiday trip to Morocco last month when he got up spontaneously with the hotel band and put together an impromptu medley of arias. I think Joseph might have invented the operatic version of Karaoke!

Ned Warwick also spoke about Joseph:

> I see Joseph in the dust and the hard sun . . . fulfilling the true meaning of life through travel, which as Robert Louis Stevenson said is to get off the feather bed of civilisation and feel the hard flintiness of the road underfoot. On his desk Oonagh found his last itinerary, for a trip in April. He wanted to take Oonagh and go to

Peru, 'Never been there,' he said simply, when I saw him last. He was full of the traveller's true excitement, he had a glint in his eye, he liked the idea of it. It was to be a round-the-world trip . . . and he had drawn in a globe's circle . . . a necklace of destinations . . . a traveller to the last.

And I couldn't help but think, when I saw it, that Joseph always had his bearings worked out . . . and if you could just lean over his shoulder and see where his compass needle was pointed . . . you had to feel that was where you should try and point yourself as well.

After the loss of so many of my loved ones, and coming so close to death myself on several occasions, I now see death as a new beginning to learning and to loving rather than a waste, a destruction or a suffering hardly to be endured. So often we forget that life is a gift and loved ones are special gifts lent to us from on High, for a time.

We unite with the spirit of our loved ones through prayer and silence. If we reach out to the Author of Love and ask His help to live without selfishness and to deepen our awareness and our compassion towards our fellow man, woman and child, then we can emerge from a sea of grief, from the inevitability of tragedy and the losing of love. It is essential to learn to laugh and love again.

As long as we are alive we have new lessons to learn. If we suffer pain and loss, courage helps more than knowledge. Human sympathy and compassion help more than courage, and prayer is very necessary to maintain peace in our hearts.

The human heart is a boundless ocean and the mind is a unique instrument. Miracles of healing take place when the heart and mind are in harmony.

The tears still flow down my cheeks, like rain on the window pane, but in the stars and the stillness of the night I see Joseph's love. He is creating a new orchestral piece to welcome me home . . . we are going to have a great party. Do join us!

CHAPTER 14

THE INNOCENCE OF LOVE

There is a way from your heart to mine
And my heart knows it, because it is clean and pure
like water.
When the water is still like a mirror, it can behold the
moon. – Rumi

Love, that wonderful gift placed in the soul, has brought me the greatest joy in life and I have been very fortunate to drink long and deep from its pure waters. If only we can recognise that its all-embracing delights are always present, we can taste the peace that they bring us.

A childhood memory which is still precious is that of the visits of my maternal grandmother: the excitement of her arrival, the quality of her whole stay, and her wonderful Victorian bonnets. I had a very special place in her heart because I was allowed to sleep with her, in her bed, and when she returned home I would accompany her across the River Shannon in the sidecar drawn by a black mare.

My grandmother was gentle and beautiful and her voice, when she read me bedtime stories, would caress me to sleep. I was six years old, and I loved her with all the innocence of a child. In my dreams – as in those of any child – my longings took me to fantastic places which either enchanted or horrified me. Enchantment can create precious moments and leave a lasting memory but darkness also inhabits the minds of children. They are often aware of evil in the form of sinister goblins and other fanciful monsters, and need a loving and understanding presence (from parents or the help of a guardian angel) to protect them.

The freedom and innocence of childhood is our essential nature and the love of a child is free of limitations. But as we grow into adulthood we begin to love in a different way. All the 'shoulds', the 'musts' and the 'oughts' can so easily obscure our path and help create seemingly deep holes into which we can fall time and again. We lose our footing and become bound by ignoring our true selves, through perpetual busyness and constantly looking outwards. Yet even in these deep holes we can still look up and see the stars (our heavenly lanterns). By catching moonbeams and lovingly playing with them, and kissing the joys as they float past, we can regain our confidence – but freedom and the strengths of innocence are found again through the restoring power of silence.

SWEET CHILD OF INNOCENCE

Oh, you sweet child of innocence
You sang a song for me
And in your smile and laughter
You set my spirit free,
You caressed away my hardships
With your gaiety and show
And in your own, but simple way
I know you let me know
That your love for me was bottomless
Over 3000 fathoms deep
And no dam could stop the love
You had laid down for me to reap.

Your mind has got one silken thread
Of a pure and magic weave
That was meant to love and glorify
Never meant to deceive
For deception has saddened many
who refuse what they receive
And they look for other answers
For they just cannot believe
That this child is just a messenger
Of a love that's rich and pure
And it's we who are too oft times sick
And too blind to see our cure.

(Tim Buckley)

INDEX

Charles, Prince of Wales 102, 103, 105, 156, 165
Chung, Lily 133

D'heurle, Geneviève 84, 88, 90
D'heurle, Michel 88, 90
Diana, Princess of Wales 14–15
  first meeting with 151
  spirituality 153, 155–6, 166
  interest in heart surgery 160–1
  friendship with 162
  death of 162, 165–8
Doherty, Maureen 149, 150
Duberry, Giselle 95, 97, 107, 109

Elizabeth II, Queen 102, 103, 104, 105

Ford, Sandra 148, 169

Johnson, Sidney 95, 97, 99, 108

Keaveny, Monsignor Patrick 68, 79, 112, 148
Khan, Hasnat 157, 158, 159

MacDonald, Margaret 133, 134, 138, 139, 147
Mairead, Sister 158
Miyake, Issey 73, 88, 150

Nedrum, Sonja 148

Paul VI, Pope 41, 64, 152
Philip, Prince 102, 105

Snowdon, Lord 88, 150
Spencer, Ignatius 167

Teresa, Mother 51, 52, 53, 155, 168
Toffolo, Joseph
  first meeting with 71–4
  trip to Oberammergau with 76–8
  trip to Nice and Italy with 86–7
  wedding to 111–112
  time in Baghdad with 114–120
  travels in Middle East with 121–7
  meeting with Princess of Wales 157
  death of 168–172

Warriner, Katherine 169
Warriner, Robert 170
Windsor, Duke of 14–15
  call to take care of 90–1
  operation in American Hospital 93–5
  nursing at home 95–102
  visit from Queen 102–6
  death of 106–110
Windsor, Duchess of
  gratitude of 98
  royal status 100
  sadness in husband's death 109–110
  quote 157

Yacoub, Sir Magdi 157, 158, 159